Clostridium difficile Infection

Editor

MARK H. WILCOX

INFECTIOUS DISEASE CLINICS OF NORTH AMERICA

www.id.theclinics.com

Consulting Editor
HELEN W. BOUCHER

March 2015 • Volume 29 • Number 1

ELSEVIER

1600 John F. Kennedy Boulevard • Suite 1800 • Philadelphia, Pennsylvania, 19103-2899.
http://www.theclinics.com

INFECTIOUS DISEASE CLINICS OF NORTH AMERICA Volume 29, Number 1
March 2015 ISSN 0891-5520, ISBN-13: 978-0-323-35657-2

Editor: Jessica McCool
Developmental Editor: Donald Mumford

Infectious Disease Clinics of North America (ISSN 0891-5520) is published in March, June, September, and December by Elsevier Inc., 360 Park Avenue South, New York, NY 10010-1710. Periodicals postage paid at New York, NY and additional mailing offices. Subscription prices are $295.00 per year for US individuals, $510.00 per year for US institutions, $145.00 per year for US students, $350.00 per year for Canadian individuals, $638.00 per year for Canadian institutions, $420.00 per year for international individuals, $638.00 per year for international institutions, and $200.00 per year for Canadian and international students. To receive student rate, orders must be accompanied by name of affiliated institution, date of term, and the *signature* of program/residency coordinator on institution letterhead. Orders will be billed at individual rate until proof of status is received. Foreign air speed delivery is included in all *Clinics* subscription prices. All prices are subject to change without notice. **POSTMASTER**: Send address changes to *Infectious Disease Clinics of North America,* Elsevier Health Sciences Division, Subcription Customer Service, 3251 Riverport Lane, Maryland Heights, MO 63043. **Customer Service: 1-800-654-2452 (US). From outside of the US and Canada, call 1-314-447-8871. Fax: 1-314-447-8029. E-mail: JournalsCustomerService-usa@elsevier.com (print support) or JournalsOnlineSupport-usa@elsevier.com (online support).**

Infectious Disease Clinics of North America is also published in Spanish by Editorial Inter-Médica, Junin 917, 1er A 1113, Buenos Aires, Argentina.

Reprints. For copies of 100 or more, of articles in this publication, please contact the Commercial Reprints Department, Elsevier Inc., 360 Park Avenue South, New York, New York 10010-1710. Tel. 212-633-3874, Fax: 212-633-3820, E-mail: reprints@elsevier.com.

Infectious Disease Clinics of North America is covered in *MEDLINE/PubMed (Index Medicus), Current Contents/Clinical Medicine, Science Citation Alert, SCISEARCH,* and *Research Alert.*

Contributors

CONSULTING EDITOR

HELEN W. BOUCHER, MD, FACP, FIDSA
Director, Infectious Diseases Fellowship Program, Division of Geographic Medicine and Infectious Diseases, Tufts Medical Center; Associate Professor of Medicine, Tufts University School of Medicine, Boston, Massachusetts

EDITOR

MARK H. WILCOX, MD, FRCPath
Professor of Medical Microbiology, Consultant Microbiologist, and Head of Microbiology, University of Leeds, Old Medical School, Leeds Teaching Hospitals, Leeds General Infirmary, Leeds, West Yorkshire, United Kingdom

AUTHORS

STEPHEN J. ALLEN, MB ChB, MRCP(UK) Paediatrics, DTM&H, MD
Professor, Department of Clinical Sciences, Liverpool School of Tropical Medicine, Liverpool, United Kingdom

MARTIJN P. BAUER, MD, PhD
Department of Infectious Diseases, Center for Infectious Diseases, Leiden University Medical Center, Leiden, The Netherlands

CAROLINE H. CHILTON, PhD
Section of Molecular Gastroenterology, Leeds Institute for Biomedical and Clinical Sciences, University of Leeds, Leeds, United Kingdom

ABHISHEK DESHPANDE, MD, PhD
Department of Infectious Diseases, Medicine Institute, Cleveland Clinic, Cleveland, Ohio

CURTIS J. DONSKEY, MD
Associate Professor of Medicine, Case Western Reserve University; Staff Physician, Infectious Diseases Section, Louis Stokes Cleveland Veterans Affairs Medical Center, Cleveland, Ohio

ERIK R. DUBBERKE, MD, MSPH
Associate Professor of Medicine, Division of Infectious Diseases, Washington University School of Medicine, St Louis, Missouri

JANE FREEMAN, PhD
Department of Microbiology, Leeds Teaching Hospitals NHS Trust, Leeds, The General Infirmary, Old Medical School, United Kingdom

DALE N. GERDING, MD
Professor, Department of Medicine, Loyola University Chicago Stritch School of Medicine, Maywood, Illinois; Research Service, Edward Hines, Jr. Veterans Affairs Hospital, Hines, Illinois

CHANDRABALI GHOSE, PhD
Aaron Diamond AIDS Research Center, New York, New York

STUART JOHNSON, MD
Professor, Loyola University Medical Center, Research Service, Hines VA Hospital, Hines, Illinois

CIARÁN P. KELLY, MD
Division of Gastroenterology, Beth Israel Deaconess Medical Center, Harvard Medical School, Boston, Massachusetts

ED J. KUIJPER, MD, PhD
Professor, Department of Medical Microbiology, Center for Infectious Diseases, Leiden University Medical Center, Leiden, The Netherlands

SIRISHA KUNDRAPU, MD
Division of Infectious Diseases and HIV Medicine, Department of Medicine, Case Western Reserve University School of Medicine, Cleveland, Ohio

JENNIE H. KWON, DO
Fellow, Division of Infectious Diseases, Washington University School of Medicine, St Louis, Missouri

FERNANDA C. LESSA, MD, MPH
Division of Healthcare Quality Promotion, National Center for Emerging and Zoonotic Infectious Diseases, Centers for Disease Control and Prevention, Atlanta, Georgia

VIVIAN G. LOO, MD, MSc
Professor of Medicine, Division of Infectious Diseases, Departments of Medicine and Microbiology, McGill University Health Centre, McGill University, Montreal, Quebec, Canada

JESSICA MARTIN, MBChB, MRCP
Academic Clinical Fellow, University of Leeds, Old Medical School, Leeds General Infirmary, Leeds, United Kingdom

TANYA M. MONAGHAN, BSc, BM, PhD, MRCP
Academic Clinical Lecturer in Gastroenterology, Biomedical Research Unit, NIHR Nottingham Digestive Diseases Centre, Nottingham University Hospitals NHS Trust, Nottingham, United Kingdom

MARGARET A. OLSEN, PhD, MPH
Associate Professor of Medicine, Divisions of Infectious Diseases and Public Health Sciences, Washington University School of Medicine, St Louis, Missouri

TIM PLANCHE, MD, FRCPath
Senior Clinical Lecturer, Honorary Consultant, and Clinical Lead for Microbiology, Division of Cellular and Molecular Medicine, Centre for Infection, University of London, St. George's Hospital, Cranmer Terrace, London, United Kingdom

KRISHNA RAO, MD
Clinical Lecturer, Division of Infectious Diseases, Department of Internal Medicine, University of Michigan School of Medicine; Veterans Affairs Ann Arbor Healthcare System, Ann Arbor, Michigan

MELINDA M. SORIANO, PharmD
Department of Pharmacy Practice, University of Illinois at Chicago, Presence Resurrection Medical Center, Chicago, Illinois

MARK H. WILCOX, MD, FRCPath
Professor of Medical Microbiology, Consultant Microbiologist, and Head of Microbiology, University of Leeds, Old Medical School, Leeds Teaching Hospitals, Leeds General Infirmary, Leeds, West Yorkshire, United Kingdom

VINCENT B. YOUNG, MD, PhD
Associate Professor, Division of Infectious Diseases, Department of Internal Medicine, Department of Microbiology and Immunology, University of Michigan School of Medicine, Ann Arbor, Michigan

Contents

when the new epidemic strain BI/NAP1/027 emerged. The article provides an overview of how understanding of *C difficile* epidemiology has rapidly evolved since its initial association with colitis in 1974. It also discusses how *C difficile* has spread across the globe, the role of asymptomatic carriers in disease transmission, the increased recognition of *C difficile* outside health care settings, the changes in epidemiology of *C difficile* infection in children, and the risk factors for disease.

Acquisition of *Clostridium difficile* spores can be followed by a spectrum of clinical outcomes ranging from asymptomatic transit through the bowel to severe colitis and death. This clinical variability is a product of bacterial virulence and host susceptibility to the pathogen. It is important to identify patients at high risk of poor outcome so that increased monitoring and optimal treatment strategies can be instigated. This article discusses the evidence linking strain type to clinical outcome, including the importance of toxin and nontoxin virulence factors. It reviews host factors and their relationship with *C difficile* infection susceptibility, recurrence, and mortality.

Accurate diagnosis of *Clostridium difficile* infection (CDI) is important not only for patient care but also for epidemiology and disease research. As it is not possible clinically to reliably differentiate CDI from other causes of health care–associated diarrhea, the laboratory confirmation of CDI is essential. Rapid commercial assays, including nucleic acid amplification tests and immunoassays for *C difficile* toxin and glutamate dehydrogenase, have largely superseded the use of older assays. Although assays that detect the presence of free *C difficile* toxin in feces are less frequently positive than tests for organism, they are preferable for the detection of CDI.

The control of *Clostridium difficile* infection is paramount. *C difficile* spores are difficult to eradicate and can survive on surfaces for prolonged periods of time. Hand washing with either plain or antimicrobial soap is effective in removing *C difficile* spores from hands. Patients should be placed in private rooms and under contact precautions to prevent transmission to other patients. Regular hospital germicides are not sporicidal and hypochlorite solutions are required for surface disinfection. In outbreak situations, a multifaceted approach is required.

Vancomycin and metronidazole were historically considered equivalent therapies for the management of *Clostridium difficile* infections (CDI); however, recent data confirm more favorable outcomes with vancomycin.

Fidaxomicin is a narrow spectrum antibiotic that has an advantage in reducing recurrence rates compared with vancomycin, possibly owing to its sparing effect on normal colonic microbiota. Data are limited for guiding management of CDI recurrences, particularly multiple recurrences. Several empiric approaches to manage these cases are reviewed.

This article discusses the use of fecal microbiota transplantation (FMT) for the treatment of recurrent *Clostridium difficile* infection (CDI). The disruption of the normal gut microbiota is central to the pathogenesis of CDI, and disruption persists in recurrent disease. The use of FMT for recurrent CDI is characterized by a high response rate and short term safety is excellent, although the long-term effects of FMT are as yet unknown.

Clostridium difficile infection (CDI) is the most common cause of infectious health care–associated diarrhea and is a major burden to patients and the health care system. The incidence and severity of CDI remain at historically high levels. This article reviews the morbidity, mortality, and costs associated with CDI.

Exposure to antibiotics is the major risk factor for *Clostridium difficile* diarrhea (CDD), suggesting that impairment of colonization resistance due to depletion of the gut flora is a significant underlying disease susceptibility factor. Many properties of probiotic organisms indicate that they may be able to replenish the depleted gut flora and restore colonization resistance. However, despite numerous clinical trials, the evidence base for probiotics in the prevention of CDD remains weak. A recent large trial of a multistrain, high-dose probiotic did not show clear evidence of efficacy. The role of probiotics in the prevention of CDD remains unclear.

Clostridium difficile is a spore-forming anaerobic gram-positive organism that is the leading cause of antibiotic-associated nosocomial infectious diarrhea in the Western world. This article describes the evolving epidemiology of *C difficile* infection (CDI) in the twenty-first century, evaluates the importance of vaccines against the disease, and defines the roles of both innate and adaptive host immune responses in CDI. The effects of passive immunotherapy and active vaccination against CDI in both humans and animals are also discussed.

In vivo and *in vitro* models are widely used to simulate *Clostridium difficile* infection (CDI). They have made considerable contributions in the study of *C difficile* pathogenesis, antibiotic predisposition to CDI, and population dynamics as well as the evaluation of new antimicrobial and immunologic therapeutics. Although CDI models have greatly increased understanding of this complicated pathogen, all have limitations in reproducing human disease, notably their inability to generate a truly reflective immune response. This review summarizes the most commonly used models of CDI and discusses their pros and cons and their predictive values in terms of clinical outcomes.

INFECTIOUS DISEASE CLINICS OF NORTH AMERICA

RELATED INTEREST

Clinics in Geriatric Medicine, February 2014 (Vol. 30, Issue 1)
Gastroenterology
Seymour Katz, *Editor*
Available at: http://www.geriatric.theclinics.com/

DOWNLOAD Free App!

Review Articles
THE CLINICS

NOW AVAILABLE FOR YOUR iPhone and iPad

Preface

Clostridium difficile Infection

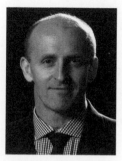

Mark H. Wilcox, MD
Editor

Clostridium difficile is the major infective cause of health care–associated diarrhea in the developed world. The epidemiology of *C difficile* infection (CDI) has been transformed in many countries by the emergence of epidemic strains, most notably the NAP1/BI/027 strain, clones of which have spread across continents. It is a disease primarily, but not exclusively, of the elderly. There is considerable excess morbidity, mortality, and cost associated with CDI, which has led to major public health campaigns in some health care systems. The Centers for Disease Control and Prevention declared *C difficile* to be one of the top three urgent infection threats in 2013. The fact that *C difficile* managed to force its way into a report dealing primarily with antibiotic resistance reflects both its frequent association with antibiotic use and the continuing high incidence of CDI in the United States.

In the current millennium, there has been an exponential increase in the number of scientific publications about *C difficile*. This reflects the substantial improvements in our understanding, in particular, of disease pathogenesis and infection control. However, there has been a focus more on understanding the pathogen and less on the host. Our quantification of the burdens imposed by CDI has also improved markedly, augmented by better disease surveillance. Until recently, there have been only modest improvements in the diagnostic options for CDI. Prophylaxis against CDI has also lagged behind, but several options are in development, notably including vaccines. The impact of CDI has stimulated considerable research into treatment options, with some recent significantly improved antimicrobial-based and microbiota-based therapeutic choices. Unusually in the field of infection, there is a healthy pipeline of novel drug and biotherapy options, which offer hope for the future.

This issue reviews the above topics and aims to provide the reader with a state-of-the-art overview of the current knowns and unknowns of this most difficult

Infect Dis Clin N Am 29 (2015) xiii–xiv
http://dx.doi.org/10.1016/j.idc.2014.12.001
0891-5520/15/$ – see front matter © 2015 Published by Elsevier Inc.

microorganism and disease. I thank all of the authors for giving their time and knowledge so generously. Most societies face marked increases in the proportion of elderly in their populations in the next 2 to 3 decades. If we do not come to terms with *C difficile*, then its threat awaits all of us.

Mark H. Wilcox, MD
Leeds Teaching Hospitals & University of Leeds
Microbiology
Old Medical School
Leeds General Infirmary
Leeds LS1 3EX, UK

E-mail address:
mark.wilcox@nhs.net

New Perspectives in *Clostridium difficile* Disease Pathogenesis

Tanya M. Monaghan, BSc, BM, PhD, MRCP

KEYWORDS

- *Clostridium difficile* • Virulence factors • Spore • Host response • Microbiota

KEY POINTS

- *Clostridium difficile* infection pathogenesis is a multifactorial process involving a complex interplay between bacterial virulence factors, the intestinal microbiota and host immune factors.
- *C difficile* spores are the principal vehicle of transmission, infection, and persistence.
- Deficiencies in innate and adaptive immune defense mechanisms affect disease outcomes.
- Inhibiting the function of the toxins, targeting specific host inflammatory pathways, and/or manipulating the intestinal microbiota may offer adjunctive treatments to current antimicrobials.

INTRODUCTION

Clostridium difficile is a gram-positive, endospore-forming, anaerobic, gastrointestinal pathogen that is the leading worldwide cause of hospital-acquired infective diarrhea.[1] *C difficile* exerts its major pathologic effects through the action of its 2 principal virulence factors, toxin A (TcdA) and toxin B (TcdB). The importance of these homologous exotoxins to *C difficile* pathogenesis is extensively supported by *in vitro* studies using epithelial cell lines derived from human colon cancer and small animal models,[2,3] as well as reports showing that *C difficile* clinical isolates lacking both toxin genes are nonpathogenic in humans and animals.[4–6] In addition to pathogenic toxin production, the composition and function of the intestinal microbiome and host immune factors have direct impacts on *C difficile* pathogenesis. This article highlights recent developments in the understanding of *C difficile* infection (CDI) pathogenesis.

Pathogenicity Locus

The genes encoding TcdA (*tcdA*) and TcdB (*tcdB*) are found on the pathogenicity locus (PaLoc), a 19.6-kb chromosomal region that also contains 3 further genes: *tcdR*,

Biomedical Research Unit, NIHR Nottingham Digestive Diseases Centre, Nottingham University Hospitals NHS Trust, Derby Road, Nottingham NG7 2UH, UK
E-mail address: tanya.monaghan@nottingham.ac.uk

Infect Dis Clin N Am 29 (2015) 1–11
http://dx.doi.org/10.1016/j.idc.2014.11.007
0891-5520/15/$ – see front matter © 2015 Elsevier Inc. All rights reserved.
id.theclinics.com

encoding an RNA polymerase sigma factor that positively regulates toxin expression[7]; *tcdC*, considered a corresponding negative regulator, although still a matter of current debate[8–11]; and *tcdE*, which is related to the bacteriophage holins.[12] In addition to *tcdR* and *tcdC*, factors outside the PaLoc, including CodY,[13] a common transcriptional regulator in gram-positive organisms, and the carbon catabolite repression system, involving the catabolite control protein, CcpA,[14] also participate in the regulation of toxin synthesis. Recent phylogenetic analyses reveal that the PaLoc resembles a mobile genetic element that has a complex evolutionary history with distinct PaLoc variants acquiring clade specificity after divergence.[15] These PacLoc variants, referred to as toxinotypes, include variants with intact genes but sequence changes, forms with truncated *tcdA*, variants of *tcdB*, and forms with *tcdC* encoding mutations and deletions.[16]

Mechanism of Action and Functional Domains of Toxin A and Toxin B

Similar to other members of the large clostridial family of toxins, TcdA and TcdB target the Rho/Ras superfamily of GTPases by irreversible modification through glucosylation at Thr-35/Th-37.[6] Because GTPases are key cellular regulatory proteins, their permanent inactivation within intoxicated epithelial cells leads to dysregulation of actin cytoskeleton and tight junction integrity, intestinal epithelial cell damage, and apoptosis by caspase activation.[6]

Both toxins are single-polypeptide chain, high-molecular-weight exotoxins arranged into large multidomain and functionally distinct structures represented schematically in **Fig. 1**. The molecular mode of action of the toxins is not completely understood. Based on current data, toxins seem to bind to an as-yet unidentified receptor and enter cells through receptor-mediated endocytosis.[17] Once inside the acidic endosomal compartment, a decrease in pH causes conformational changes within the toxin, allowing pore formation and subsequent translocation of the catalytic glucosyltransferase domain across the endosomal membrane. Knowledge of exactly how this process occurs and which regions of the translocation domain are critical for this process is starting to emerge. Recent findings have uncovered the pore-forming hotspot of the TcdB translocation domain, clustered between amino acid residues 1035 and 1107, which, when individually mutated, reduces cellular toxicity by greater than 1000-fold.[18] Release of the glucosyltransferase enzymatic moiety into the cytosol occurs by an autoproteolytic cleavage event, which is thought to involve exposure to the cysteine protease domain and requires inositol hexakisphosphate (InsP6).[19,20]

The relative importance of each toxin in disease pathogenesis is still a matter of debate. Both toxins seem to be lethal in animal challenge models, supported further by *C difficile* genetic manipulation studies reporting that TcdA⁻TcdB⁺ and TcdA⁺TcdB⁻ mutants of *C difficile* caused disease in hamsters.[21,22] Nevertheless, an earlier report generating equivalent mutants in the same *C difficile* strain found that only TcdB was essential for virulence, whereas TcdA was dispensable.[23] In support of the dominant role of TcdB, all naturally occurring pathogenic strains produce TcdB (but not necessarily TcdA), suggesting that TcdB may play the dominant role in human infection.[23–25]

Other Clostridium difficile Virulence Components

Some *C difficile* strains (eg, 027 and 078 ribotypes) also produce an adenosine diphosphate ribosyltransferase toxin, commonly referred to as *C difficile* binary toxin (CDT). This toxin is composed of an enzymatically active A component (CDTa), which causes ADP-ribosylation of G-actin, and a cell-binding and translocation B

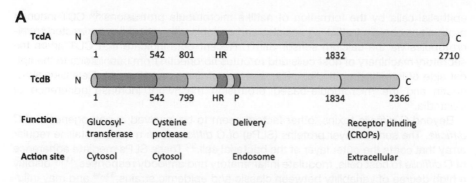

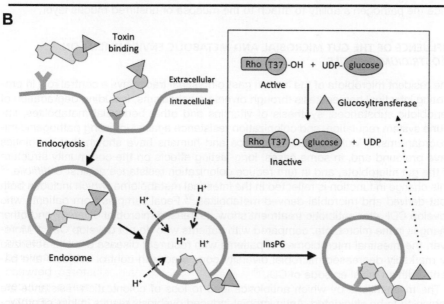

Fig. 1. (A) Structure of TcdA and TcdB. TcdA and TcdB are large multidomain proteins consisting of an N-terminal catalytic domain with glucosyltransferase activity, a delivery or pore-forming domain, a cysteine protease region involved in toxin entry into target epithelial cells, and a C-terminal host cell–binding region consisting of combined repetitive oligopeptide repeats (CROPs). The P zone represents the hydrophobic region of the delivery domain that has been proposed to form the *C difficile* TcdB translocation pore, clustered between amino acids 1035 and 1107. (B) Mechanism of action of TcdA and TcdB. Toxin binds to the surface of epithelial cells using the C-terminal receptor-binding domain. Binding triggers toxin internalization via clathrin-mediated endocytosis. Acidification of the endosome creates a pore that is thought to enable translocation of the glucosyltransferase domain into the cytosol. Exposure of the cysteine protease domain to inositol hexakisphosphate (InsP6) activates an autoproteolytic cleavage event, resulting in the release of the glucosyltransferase domain into the cytosol. The glucosyltransferase domain transfers a glucose moiety from the donor substrate uridine diphosphate (UDP)-glucose to a threonine residue (Thr-37 in RhoA), thereby inactivating intracellular Rho and Ras family GTPases.

component, CDTb.[26] The CDTb component is activated by serine proteases and binds to a lipolysis-stimulated lipoprotein receptor.[27] Although the biological significance of CDT during infection remains unclear, *in vitro* studies show that purified CDT is toxic to Vero cells and may increase adherence of *C difficile* to intestinal epithelial cells by the formation of netlike microtubule protrusions.[28] CDT-induced protrusions contain trafficking vesicles and endoplasmic reticulum, connected to microtubules via the calcium sensor Stim1. Recent data indicate that CDT alters the secretory machinery of host cells and reroutes fibronectin from basolateral to the apical side of intestinal epithelial cells, where protrusions are formed. Released fibronectin and the microtubule-based protrusion meshwork increase adherence of clostridia.[29]

Beyond *C difficile* toxins, other factors seem to be involved in pathogenesis of *C difficile*. The surface layer proteins (SLPs) of *C difficile* form a paracrystalline regular array that coats the outer layer of the bacterial cell.[30] These SLPs mediate adherence of *C difficile* to host cells, modulate inflammatory and antibody responses,[31,32] display a high degree of variability between classic and epidemic strains,[33,34] and may influence the pathogen's ability to attach to the mucosa or unstirred mucus layer.

INFLUENCE OF THE GUT MICROBIAL AND METABOLIC ENVIRONMENT ON *CLOSTRIDIUM DIFFICILE*

The resident microbiota of the human gastrointestinal tract plays a central role in promoting intestinal homeostasis through diverse mechanisms, including degradation of xenobiotic substances, synthesis of vitamins and other beneficial metabolites, immune system regulation, and colonization resistance against invading pathogenic microorganisms.[35] Multiple studies in mice and humans have shown that antibiotics have profound and, in some cases, long-lasting effects on the community structure of the gut microbiota, and in turn reduce colonization resistance against *C difficile*.[36] This change in function is reflected in the intestinal metabolome, which includes both host-derived and microbial-derived metabolites.[37] Fecal samples from patients who develop CDI after antibiotic treatment show decreased microbial diversity and other changes in the microbiota, compared with patients who do not develop CDI.[38] Moreover, the intestinal microbiomes of patients with recurrent disease are characterized by markedly decreased microbial diversity compared with control subjects and patients with an initial episode of CDI.[39]

The mechanisms by which antibiotics lead to loss of colonization resistance are beginning to be elucidated. Antimicrobial-induced dysbiosis results in loss of protective toll-like receptor (TLR) signaling, accumulation of proinflammatory T helper 17 T cells, and increased epithelial permeability.[40] Subsequent infection with *C difficile* leads to additional toxin-mediated epithelial injury, access to lamina propria immune cells, and perpetuation of the proinflammatory response.[41]

In murine infection models, dysbiosis can promote *C difficile* transmission by creating a supershedder phenotype, allowing *C difficile* to transmit very effectively.[42,43] On closer inspection, the microbiota from these supershedders produced fewer short-chain fatty acids compared with naive and clindamycin-treated controls.[42] Short-chain fatty acids, including acetate, butyrate, and propionate, are important nutrients for mucosal and immune homeostasis.[44] Further evidence indicates that the metabolic environment of the murine intestinal tract following antibiotic treatment is enriched with primary bile acids and carbohydrates that support germination and growth of *C difficile in vitro* and *ex vivo*.[45] Another study suggests that sialic acids are increasingly released by gut commensals after antibiotic treatment, possibly enhancing *C difficile* growth.[46]

Underscoring the significant impact of dysbiosis on *C difficile*–mediated disease, there is now clear compelling evidence to suggest that therapeutic restoration of the diversity of the intestinal microbiota can restore colonization resistance. Patients with recurrent CDI can eliminate *C difficile* after receiving a healthy microbiota through strategies such as fecal microbiota transplantation.[47,48]

ROLE OF THE HOST IMMUNE RESPONSE IN *CLOSTRIDIUM DIFFICILE* INFECTION

Following CDI, both the innate and adaptive arms of the immune system are activated, suggesting that host immune responses are important determinants of disease pathogenesis.[32,49,50]

Innate Immune Responses

The early pathogenesis of CDI is predominantly characterized by acute intestinal inflammation that is mediated by the inducible innate immune response. *C difficile* is able to subvert the normally protective effects afforded by the mucus layer overlying the epithelium by downregulating mucin exocytosis from mucin-producing human colonic epithelial cells during infection.[51,52] However, host epithelial-derived antimicrobial peptides, defensins, and cathelicidins can significantly reduce *C difficile* toxin–induced tissue damage and inflammation.[53,54]

In vitro studies have shown that *C difficile* TcdA acts rapidly on intestinal epithelial cells, causing cellular rounding, detachment, apoptosis, and the secretion of proinflammatory cytokines, including the potent neutrophil chemoattractant interleukin (IL)-8.[55] Neutrophils contribute significantly to tissue damage, because they contain a potent arsenal of oxidants and proteases in azurophilic granules.[56] Following the loss of epithelial cells, exposure of lamina propria cells to TcdA *in vitro* induces apoptosis in macrophages, eosinophils, and T cells,[57] which trigger dissemination of the inflammatory cascade via further release of proinflammatory cytokines and chemokines including IL-12, IL-18, interferon gamma, IL-1β, tumor necrosis factor alpha, macrophage inflammatory protein (MIP) 1 alpha, MIP-2, IL-8, and leptin.[58,59]

In addition, *C difficile* can activate both surface and intracellular innate immune sensors, including the IL-1β/inflammasome, TLR4, TLR5, and nucleotide-binding oligomerization domain 1 signaling pathways.[60–63] Nitric oxide has also emerged as an important innate immune defense mechanism against *C difficile*, ameliorating disease in murine models by inhibiting neutrophil migration, hypoxia-inducible factor 1-alpha, and inflammasome activity, as well as directly inhibiting the potency of the toxins.[64] The protective effects of nitric oxide signal transduction seem in large part to be mediated by pleiotropic S-nitrosylation signals that result from increased nitric oxide synthase 2A activity.[65]

Both toxins may also lead to activation, degranulation, and the release of inflammatory mediators from mast cells[66] and can stimulate a strong neuroinflammatory response via secretion of various neuropeptides and neuroimmune signals.[32] Intestinal dendritic cells also respond to *C difficile* antigens, including SLPs and *C difficile* toxins, by promoting the release of regulatory and antiinflammatory cytokines such as IL-10, IL-23, and IL-4. These cytokines initiate cellular repair processes, dampen the inflammatory response, and activate regulatory T cells and B lymphocytes to promote the protective adaptive antibody response.[60,67,68]

Adaptive Immune Responses

Reports from multiple animal models and human studies clearly indicate that humoral immune responses to TcdA and TcdB influence the outcomes of CDI.[49] Most notably, symptomless carriers of toxigenic *C difficile* and those with a single episode of CDI without recurrence show more robust anti-TcdA immunoglobulin (Ig) G immune responses than patients with symptomatic and recurrent disease.[49] More recently, several reports have observed an association between higher levels of anti-TcdB antibodies and lower levels of disease.[69–72] It is not known whether this is caused by a central role of anti-TcdB in preventing recurrence or whether TcdB is more immunogenic than TcdA in humans.[73] There is also evidence suggesting that sera responses may be nondurable[74] or weaker in the elderly,[71,75,76] observations that are consistent with the phenomenon known as immune senescence.[77]

The importance of the adaptive immune response in modulating CDI outcomes is perhaps best highlighted by the number of experimental vaccines currently under development.[78] Furthermore, a phase II human trial showed a large (72%) reduction in C difficile recurrence rate in subjects given a mixture of 2 neutralizing human IgG1 anti-TcdA and TcdB antibodies.[79]

CLOSTRIDIUM DIFFICILE SPORULATION AND GERMINATION

C difficile spores are the main vehicle of persistence (CDI recurrence) and transmission of strains.[80] This finding has been supported by recent studies in which a mutant strain of C difficile, unable to produce the Spo0A protein (a transcriptional regulatory protein essential for the initiation of sporulation), did not persist or transmit disease in a mouse model.[81] C difficile spores are metabolically dormant and therefore intrinsically resistant to antibiotics[82] and attacks from the host's immune system,[83,84] and once shed into the environment are resistant to disinfectants.[85]

In order to initiate infection in the host, ingested C difficile spores must germinate into toxin-expressing vegetative cells in the intestinal tract.[86] C difficile spores germinate in response to specific bile salts (cholate, taurocholate, glycocholate, and deoxycholate) and L-glycine acts as a cogerminant.[87–89] These salts bind to CspC, a catalytically dead serine protease that acts as a germinant receptor.[90] New evidence points to strain-to-strain variability in the germination response to bile salts, with variation also observed in the germination efficiency of C difficile spores.[80]

SUMMARY

Although knowledge of the mechanisms underlying C difficile pathogenesis has increased markedly in recent years, many important outstanding questions remain. For example, what are the human receptors for TcdA and TcdB; which cells do they target in vivo; how significant are the roles of binary toxin and nontoxin components in determining bacterial virulence; how do innate immune responses influence disease progression and outcome in C difficile; and which factors are involved in modulating C difficile spore resistance, germination, and sporulation? Further advances in murine models of infection, microbial culturing, DNA sequencing technologies, gene-editing tools, mucosal immunology, and in vivo–like three-dimensional intestinal organoid platforms[3,91–96] should help facilitate the development of novel and more targeted therapies for this difficult pathogen.

REFERENCES

1. Clements AC, Magalhaes RJ, Tatem AJ, et al. Clostridium difficile PCR ribotype 027: assessing the risks of further worldwide spread. Lancet Infect Dis 2010; 10:395–404.
2. Best EL, Freeman J, Wilcox MH. Models for the study of Clostridium difficile infection. Gut Microbes 2012;3:145–67.

3. Hutton ML, Mackin KE, Chakravorty A, et al. Small animal models for the study of *Clostridium difficile* disease pathogenesis. FEMS Microbiol Lett 2014;352:140–9.
4. Elliott B, Chang BJ, Golledge CL, et al. *Clostridium difficile*-associated diarrhoea. Intern Med J 2007;37:561–8.
5. Kelly CP, Pothoulakis C, LaMont JT. *Clostridium difficile* colitis. N Engl J Med 1994;330:257–62.
6. Voth DE, Ballard JD. *Clostridium difficile* toxins: mechanism of action and role in disease. Clin Microbiol Rev 2005;18:247–63.
7. Mani N, Dupuy B. Regulation of toxin synthesis in *Clostridium difficile* by an alternative RNA polymerase sigma factor. Proc Natl Acad Sci U S A 2001;98: 5844–9.
8. Hundsberger T, Braun V, Weidmann M, et al. Transcription analysis of the genes tcdA-E of the pathogenicity locus of *Clostridium difficile*. Eur J Biochem 1997; 244:735–42.
9. Matamouros S, England P, Dupuy B. *Clostridium difficile* toxin expression is inhibited by the novel regulator TcdC. Mol Microbiol 2007;64:1274–88.
10. Cartman ST, Kelly ML, Heeg D, et al. Precise manipulation of the *Clostridium difficile* chromosome reveals a lack of association between the tcdC genotype and toxin production. Appl Environ Microbiol 2012;78:4683–90.
11. Bakker D, Smits WK, Kuijper EJ, et al. TcdC does not significantly repress toxin expression in *Clostridium difficile* 630DeltaErm. PLoS One 2012;7:e43247.
12. Tan KS, Wee BY, Song KP. Evidence for holin function of tcdE gene in the pathogenicity of *Clostridium difficile*. J Med Microbiol 2001;50:613–9.
13. Dineen SS, Villapakkam AC, Nordman JT, et al. Repression of *Clostridium difficile* toxin gene expression by CodY. Mol Microbiol 2007;66:206–19.
14. Antunes A, Martin-Verstraete I, Dupuy B. CcpA-mediated repression of *Clostridium difficile* toxin gene expression. Mol Microbiol 2011;79:882–99.
15. Dingle KE, Elliott B, Robinson E, et al. Evolutionary history of the *Clostridium difficile* pathogenicity locus. Genome Biol Evol 2014;6:36–52.
16. Hunt JJ, Ballard JD. Variations in virulence and molecular biology among emerging strains of *Clostridium difficile*. Microbiol Mol Biol Rev 2013;77: 567–81.
17. Papatheodorou P, Zamboglou C, Genisyuerek S, et al. Clostridial glucosylating toxins enter cells via clathrin-mediated endocytosis. PLoS One 2010;5:e10673.
18. Zhang Z, Park M, Tam J, et al. Translocation domain mutations affecting cellular toxicity identify the *Clostridium difficile* toxin B pore. Proc Natl Acad Sci U S A 2014; 111:3721–6.
19. Egerer M, Giesemann T, Jank T, et al. Auto ootalytic cleavage of *Clostridium difficile* toxins A and B depends on cysteine protease activity. J Biol Chem 2007;282: 25314–21.
20. Pruitt RN, Chagot B, Cover M, et al. Structure-function analysis of inositol hexakisphosphate-induced autoprocessing in *Clostridium difficile* toxin A. J Biol Chem 2009;284:21934–40.
21. Kuehne SA, Cartman ST, Heap JT, et al. The role of toxin A and toxin B in *Clostridium difficile* infection. Nature 2010;467:711–3.
22. Kuehne SA, Cartman ST, Minton NP. Both, toxin A and toxin B, are important in *Clostridium difficile* infection. Gut Microbes 2011;2:252–5.
23. Lyras D, O'Connor JR, Howarth PM, et al. Toxin B is essential for virulence of *Clostridium difficile*. Nature 2009;458:1176–9.
24. Loo VG, Bourgault AM, Poirier L, et al. Host and pathogen factors for *Clostridium difficile* infection and colonization. N Engl J Med 2011;365:1693–703.

25. Steele J, Mukherjee J, Parry N, et al. Antibody against TcdB, but not TcdA, prevents development of gastrointestinal and systemic *Clostridium difficile* disease. J Infect Dis 2013;207:323–30.

26. Gerding DN, Johnson S, Rupnik M, et al. *Clostridium difficile* binary toxin CDT: mechanism, epidemiology, and potential clinical importance. Gut Microbes 2014;5:15–27.

27. Papatheodorou P, Carette JE, Bell GW, et al. Lipolysis-stimulated lipoprotein receptor (LSR) is the host receptor for the binary toxin *Clostridium difficile* transferase (CDT). Proc Natl Acad Sci U S A 2011;108:16422–7.

28. Schwan C, Stecher B, Tzivelekidis T, et al. *Clostridium difficile* toxin CDT induces formation of microtubule-based protrusions and increases adherence of bacteria. PLoS Pathog 2009;5:e1000626.

29. Schwan C, Kruppke AS, Nolke T, et al. *Clostridium difficile* toxin CDT hijacks microtubule organization and reroutes vesicle traffic to increase pathogen adherence. Proc Natl Acad Sci U S A 2014;111:2313–8.

30. Fagan RP, Albesa-Jove D, Qazi O, et al. Structural insights into the molecular organization of the S-layer from *Clostridium difficile*. Mol Microbiol 2009;71:1308–22.

31. Vedantam G, Clark A, Chu M, et al. *Clostridium difficile* infection: toxins and nontoxin virulence factors, and their contributions to disease establishment and host response. Gut Microbes 2012;3:121–34.

32. Madan R, Jr WA. Immune responses to *Clostridium difficile* infection. Trends Mol Med 2012;18:658–66.

33. Rupnik M, Wilcox MH, Gerding DN. *Clostridium difficile* infection: new developments in epidemiology and pathogenesis. Nat Rev Microbiol 2009;7:526–36.

34. Dingle KE, Didelot X, Ansari MA, et al. Recombinational switching of the *Clostridium difficile* S-layer and a novel glycosylation gene cluster revealed by large-scale whole-genome sequencing. J Infect Dis 2013;207:675–86.

35. Walker AW, Lawley TD. Therapeutic modulation of intestinal dysbiosis. Pharmacol Res 2013;69:75–86.

36. Britton RA, Young VB. Role of the intestinal microbiota in resistance to colonization by *Clostridium difficile*. Gastroenterology 2014;146:1547–53.

37. Theriot CM, Young VB. Microbial and metabolic interactions between the gastrointestinal tract and infection. Gut Microbes 2014;5:86–95.

38. Peterfreund GL, Vandivier LE, Sinha R, et al. Succession in the gut microbiome following antibiotic and antibody therapies for *Clostridium difficile*. PLoS One 2012;7:e46966.

39. Chang JY, Antonopoulos DA, Kalra A, et al. Decreased diversity of the fecal microbiome in recurrent *Clostridium difficile*-associated diarrhea. J Infect Dis 2008; 197:435–8.

40. Littman DR, Pamer EG. Role of the commensal microbiota in normal and pathogenic host immune responses. Cell Host Microbe 2011;10:311–23.

41. Solomon K. The host immune response to *Clostridium difficile* infection. Ther Adv Infect Dis 2013;1:19–35.

42. Lawley TD, Clare S, Walker AW, et al. Targeted restoration of the intestinal microbiota with a simple, defined bacteriotherapy resolves relapsing *Clostridium difficile* disease in mice. PLoS Pathog 2012;8:e1002995.

43. Lawley TD, Clare S, Walker AW, et al. Antibiotic treatment of *Clostridium difficile* carrier mice triggers a supershedder state, spore-mediated transmission, and severe disease in immunocompromised hosts. Infect Immun 2009;77:3661–9.

44. Maslowski KM, Mackay CR. Diet, gut microbiota and immune responses. Nat Immunol 2011;12:5–9.

45. Theriot CM, Koenigsknecht MJ, Carlson PE Jr, et al. Antibiotic-induced shifts in the mouse gut microbiome and metabolome increase susceptibility to *Clostridium difficile* infection. Nat Commun 2014;5:3114.
46. Ng KM, Ferreyra JA, Higginbottom SK, et al. Microbiota-liberated host sugars facilitate post-antibiotic expansion of enteric pathogens. Nature 2013;502:96–9.
47. Dodin M, Katz DE. Faecal microbiota transplantation for *Clostridium difficile* infection. Int J Clin Pract 2014;68:363–8.
48. Borody TJ, Brandt LJ, Paramsothy S. Therapeutic faecal microbiota transplantation: current status and future developments. Curr Opin Gastroenterol 2014;30: 97–105.
49. Kelly CP, Kyne L. The host immune response to *Clostridium difficile*. J Med Microbiol 2011;60:1070–9.
50. Shen A, Lupardus PJ, Gersch MM, et al. Defining an allosteric circuit in the cysteine protease domain of *Clostridium difficile* toxins. Nat Struct Mol Biol 2011;18:364–71.
51. Branka JE, Vallette G, Jarry A, et al. Early functional effects of *Clostridium difficile* toxin A on human colonocytes. Gastroenterology 1997;112:1887–94.
52. Corfield AP, Myerscough N, Longman R, et al. Mucins and mucosal protection in the gastrointestinal tract: new prospects for mucins in the pathology of gastrointestinal disease. Gut 2000;47:589–94.
53. Hing TC, Ho S, Shih DQ, et al. The antimicrobial peptide cathelicidin modulates *Clostridium difficile*-associated colitis and toxin A-mediated enteritis in mice. Gut 2013;62:1295–305.
54. Giesemann T, Guttenberg G, Aktories K. Human alpha-defensins inhibit *Clostridium difficile* toxin B. Gastroenterology 2008;134:2049–58.
55. Mahida YR, Makh S, Hyde S, et al. Effect of *Clostridium difficile* toxin A on human intestinal epithelial cells: induction of interleukin 8 production and apoptosis after cell detachment. Gut 1996;38:337–47.
56. Kelly CP, Becker S, Linevsky JK, et al. Neutrophil recruitment in *Clostridium difficile* toxin A enteritis in the rabbit. J Clin Invest 1994;93:1257–65.
57. Mahida YR, Galvin A, Makh S, et al. Effect of *Clostridium difficile* toxin A on human colonic lamina propria cells: early loss of macrophages followed by T-cell apoptosis. Infect Immun 1998;66:5462–9.
58. Mykoniatis A, Anton PM, Wlk M, et al. Leptin mediates *Clostridium difficile* toxin A-induced enteritis in mice. Gastroenterology 2003;124:683–91.
59. Ishida Y, Maegawa T, Kondo T, et al. Essential involvement of IFN-gamma in *Clostridium difficile* toxin A-induced enteritis. J Immunol 2004;172:3018–25.
60. Ryan A, Lynch M, Smith SM, et al. A role for TLR4 in *Clostridium difficile* infection and the recognition of surface layer proteins. PLoS Pathog 2011;7:e1002076.
61. Jarchum I, Liu M, Lipuma L, et al. Toll-like receptor 5 stimulation protects mice from acute *Clostridium difficile* colitis. Infect Immun 2011;79:1498–503.
62. Hasegawa M, Yamazaki T, Kamada N, et al. Nucleotide-binding oligomerization domain 1 mediates recognition of *Clostridium difficile* and induces neutrophil recruitment and protection against the pathogen. J Immunol 2011;186:4872–80.
63. Ng J, Hirota SA, Gross O, et al. *Clostridium difficile* toxin-induced inflammation and intestinal injury are mediated by the inflammasome. Gastroenterology 2010;139:542–52, 52.e1–3.
64. Savidge TC, Urvil P, Oezguen N, et al. Host S-nitrosylation inhibits clostridial small molecule-activated glucosylating toxins. Nat Med 2011;17:1136–41.
65. Peniche AG, Savidge TC, Dann SM. Recent insights into *Clostridium difficile* pathogenesis. Curr Opin Infect Dis 2013;26:447–53.

66. Meyer GK, Neetz A, Brandes G, et al. *Clostridium difficile* toxins A and B directly stimulate human mast cells. Infect Immun 2007;75:3868–76.
67. Steele J, Chen K, Sun X, et al. Systemic dissemination of *Clostridium difficile* toxins A and B is associated with severe, fatal disease in animal models. J Infect Dis 2012;205:384–91.
68. Bianco M, Fedele G, Quattrini A, et al. Immunomodulatory activities of surface-layer proteins obtained from epidemic and hypervirulent *Clostridium difficile* strains. J Med Microbiol 2011;60:1162–7.
69. Wullt M, Noren T, Ljungh A, et al. IgG antibody response to toxins A and B in patients with *Clostridium difficile* infection. Clin Vaccine Immunol 2012;19:1552–4.
70. Aronsson B, Granstrom M, Mollby R, et al. Serum antibody response to *Clostridium difficile* toxins in patients with *Clostridium difficile* diarrhoea. Infection 1985;13:97–101.
71. Monaghan TM, Robins A, Knox A, et al. Circulating antibody and memory B-Cell responses to *C. difficile* toxins A and B in patients with *C. difficile*-associated diarrhoea, inflammatory bowel disease and cystic fibrosis. PLoS One 2013;8:e74452.
72. Leav BA, Blair B, Leney M, et al. Serum anti-toxin B antibody correlates with protection from recurrent *Clostridium difficile* infection (CDI). Vaccine 2010;28:965–9.
73. Humphreys DP, Wilcox MH. Antibodies for the treatment of *Clostridium difficile* infection. Clin Vaccine Immunol 2014;21(7):913–23.
74. Lishman AH, Al-Jumaili IJ, Record CO. Antitoxin production in antibiotic-associated colitis? J Clin Pathol 1981;34:414–5.
75. Bacon AE 3rd, Fekety R. Immunoglobulin G directed against toxins A and B of *Clostridium difficile* in the general population and patients with antibiotic-associated diarrhea. Diagn Microbiol Infect Dis 1994;18:205–9.
76. Nakamura S, Mikawa M, Nakashio S, et al. Isolation of *Clostridium difficile* from the feces and the antibody in sera of young and elderly adults. Microbiol Immunol 1981;25:345–51.
77. Kovaiou RD, Herndler-Brandstetter D, Grubeck-Loebenstein B. Age-related changes in immunity: implications for vaccination in the elderly. Expert Rev Mol Med 2007;9:1–17.
78. Leuzzi R, Adamo R, Scarselli M. Vaccines against *Clostridium difficile*. Hum Vaccin Immunother 2014;10:1466–77.
79. Lowy I, Molrine DC, Leav BA, et al. Treatment with monoclonal antibodies against *Clostridium difficile* toxins. N Engl J Med 2010;362:197–205.
80. Barra-Carrasco J, Paredes-Sabja D. *Clostridium difficile* spores: a major threat to the hospital environment. Future Microbiol 2014;9:475–86.
81. Deakin LJ, Clare S, Fagan RP, et al. The *Clostridium difficile* spo0A gene is a persistence and transmission factor. Infect Immun 2012;80:2704–11.
82. Baines SD, O'Connor R, Saxton K, et al. Activity of vancomycin against epidemic *Clostridium difficile* strains in a human gut model. J Antimicrob Chemother 2009; 63:520–5.
83. Paredes-Sabja D, Cofre-Araneda G, Brito-Silva C, et al. *Clostridium difficile* spore-macrophage interactions: spore survival. PLoS One 2012;7:e43635.
84. Paredes-Sabja D, Sarker MR. Interactions between *Clostridium perfringens* spores and Raw 264.7 macrophages. Anaerobe 2012;18:148–56.
85. Ali S, Moore G, Wilson AP. Spread and persistence of *Clostridium difficile* spores during and after cleaning with sporicidal disinfectants. J Hosp Infect 2011;79: 97–8.
86. Paredes-Sabja D, Shen A, Sorg JA. *Clostridium difficile* spore biology: sporulation, germination, and spore structural proteins. Trends Microbiol 2014;22(7):406–16.

87. Sorg JA, Sonenshein AL. Bile salts and glycine as cogerminants for *Clostridium difficile* spores. J Bacteriol 2008;190:2505–12.
88. Wheeldon LJ, Worthington T, Lambert PA. Histidine acts as a co-germinant with glycine and taurocholate for *Clostridium difficile* spores. J Appl Microbiol 2011; 110(4):987–94.
89. Howerton A, Ramirez N, Abel-Santos E. Mapping interactions between germinants and *Clostridium difficile* spores. J Bacteriol 2011;193:274–82.
90. Francis MB, Allen CA, Shrestha R, et al. Bile acid recognition by the *Clostridium difficile* germinant receptor, CspC, is important for establishing infection. PLoS Pathog 2013;9:e1003356.
91. Nagarajan K, Loh KC. Molecular biology-based methods for quantification of bacteria in mixed culture: perspectives and limitations. Appl Microbiol Biotechnol 2014;98(16):6907–19.
92. Solomon KV, Haitjema CH, Thompson DA, et al. Extracting data from the muck: deriving biological insight from complex microbial communities and non-model organisms with next generation sequencing. Curr Opin Biotechnol 2014;28C: 103–10.
93. Cho SW, Kim S, Kim JM, et al. Targeted genome engineering in human cells with the Cas9 RNA-guided endonuclease. Nat Biotechnol 2013;31:230–2.
94. Buffie CG, Pamer EG. Microbiota-mediated colonization resistance against intestinal pathogens. Nat Rev Immunol 2013;13:790–801.
95. Leushacke M, Barker N. Ex vivo culture of the intestinal epithelium: strategies and applications. Gut 2014;63:1345–54.
96. Foulke-Abel J, In J, Kovbasnjuk O, et al. Human enteroids as an ex-vivo model of host-pathogen interactions in the gastrointestinal tract. Exp Biol Med (Maywood) 2014;239(9):1124–34.

Colonization Versus Carriage of *Clostridium difficile*

Curtis J. Donskey, MD[a],*, Sirisha Kundrapu, MD[b], Abhishek Deshpande, MD, PhD[c]

KEYWORDS

- *Clostridium difficile* • Colonization • Antibiotic • Transmission

KEY POINTS

- Asymptomatic carriage of *Clostridium difficile* is common in health care facilities and the community.
- Detection of *C difficile* in stool may represent transient carriage, low-level colonization, or high-level colonization with frequent skin and environmental shedding.
- There is evidence that asymptomatic carriers may contribute to transmission, and studies are needed to determine whether interventions focused on carriers will reduce rates of *C difficile* infection.

INTRODUCTION

Many people acquiring colonization with toxigenic strains of *Clostridium difficile* become asymptomatic carriers.[1–6] In addition, many patients with *C difficile* infection (CDI) become asymptomatic carriers after successful treatment, with continued shedding of spores.[7,8] These asymptomatic carriers represent a large potential reservoir for transmission. However, current control efforts focus almost entirely on symptomatic patients because the role of asymptomatic carriers in transmission has been uncertain. However, control measures focused on symptomatic patients have often proved to be ineffective during the past decade when infection rates have increased greatly in the setting of large outbreaks of the 027/BI/NAP1 strain.

Findings from recent studies have stimulated renewed interest in asymptomatic carriers of *C difficile* as a potential source of transmission. However, several areas of

This work was supported by the Department of Veterans Affairs.
[a] Infectious Diseases Section, Louis Stokes Cleveland Veterans Affairs Medical Center, 10701 East Boulevard, Cleveland, OH 44106, USA; [b] Division of Infectious Diseases & HIV Medicine, Department of Medicine, Case Western Reserve University School of Medicine, 10900 Euclid Avenue, Cleveland, OH 44106, USA; [c] Department of Infectious Diseases, Medicine Institute, Cleveland Clinic, 9500 Euclid Avenue, Cleveland, OH 44106, USA
* Corresponding author.
E-mail address: curtisd123@yahoo.com

uncertainty require clarification before control measures focused on carriers are likely to become routine. In this article, findings from studies involving animal models, healthy volunteers, and patients are used to discuss general concepts regarding the pathogenesis and epidemiology of *C difficile* colonization. The evidence that asymptomatic carriers shed spores and contribute to transmission is examined. In addition, practical questions that must be considered in future interventions focused on carriers are discussed.

EPIDEMIOLOGY

Asymptomatic carriage of toxigenic and nontoxigenic *C difficile* is common in health care facilities. In hospitals, the prevalence or incidence of asymptomatic carriage has ranged from 7% to 18%.[2–6,9–17] **Table 1** shows findings from 6 studies that included rectal or stool cultures on admission and during hospitalization. There are several notable findings. First, asymptomatic carriage is often present on admission, with prior hospitalization being a common risk factor.[2–6,15] Other recent studies have shown frequent asymptomatic carriage on hospital admission.[9,17] Second, persistence of positive cultures was common. Third, Clabots and colleagues[3] showed that acquisition increased with increasing length of stay, increasing to 50% with stays of greater than 4 weeks. In addition, Loo and colleagues[6] found that antibiotic exposure was associated with CDI, but not asymptomatic carriage; asymptomatic carriage was associated with recent hospitalization, chemotherapy, and acid-suppressive medications. Alasmari and colleagues[9] similarly reported that carriage on admission was not associated with recent antimicrobial exposures.

Asymptomatic carriage of *C difficile* is also common in long-term care facilities (LTCFs),[18,19] including on admission.[20] In an outbreak setting, Riggs and colleagues[18] found that 51% of asymptomatic patients on 2 LTCF wards were colonized with toxigenic *C difficile*, and 37% carried epidemic NAP1/027/BI strains. Asymptomatic carriers outnumbered patients with CDI 7 to 1. Antibiotic exposure and recent CDI were risk factors for asymptomatic carriage.

The frequency of asymptomatic carriage in community-dwelling individuals is typically lower than in health care settings.[21–23] Rea and colleagues[23] reported *C difficile* carriage in 2% of elderly people in the community versus 10% in the community with outpatient health care exposures and 21% in hospital or LTCF settings. Galdys and colleagues[24] reported that 7 of 106 (7%) healthy adults with no recent health care exposures had toxigenic *C difficile* in stool. Three of 9 stool specimens tested positive with a commercial nucleic acid amplification test, raising concern that carriers in the community could test falsely positive for *C difficile* if tested for CDI when they have other causes of diarrhea.

A variety of factors may contribute to the infrequency of asymptomatic carriage in community-dwelling adults. Exposure to *C difficile* may occur less frequently in many community settings, or strain types encountered in the community might be less likely to establish persistent colonization. However, studies of healthy adults receiving antibiotics suggest that exposure is common in outpatient settings. As shown in **Fig. 1**, healthy community-dwelling subjects receiving cefixime or cefpodoxime frequently acquired *C difficile* colonization, whereas controls did not.[25] Thus, infrequent recovery of *C difficile* in community versus health care facility surveys may be related to lower levels of antibiotic exposure in the community.

COLONIZATION VERSUS TRANSIENT CARRIAGE

The terms colonization and carriage are often used interchangeably in epidemiologic studies. However, terminology related to colonization is not standardized. In intestinal

Table 1
Asymptomatic carriage and CDI on hospital admission versus acquired during hospitalization

Ref. #	2	3	4	5	6	15
Setting	Medical Ward, n (%)	Medical-Surgical Ward, n (%)	3 ICUs/2 Medical-Surgical Wards, n (%)	2 Medical Wards, n (%)	6 Hospitals, n (%)	Medical Wards, n (%)
C difficile positive on admission	29 of 428 (7)	65 of 634 (10)[a]	55 of 496 (11)[b]	37 of 271 (14)	—	16 of 168 (10)[c]
Asymptomatic carriage	17 of 29 (59)	61 of 65 (94)	44 of 55 (80)[d]	19 of 37 (51)[e]	184 of 4143 (4)	16 of 168 (10
CDI	12 of 29 (41)	4 of 65 (6)	11 of 55 (20)	18 of 37 (49)	[f]	Excluded
C difficile acquired during hospital stay	83 of 399 (21)	54 of 569 (10)	34 of 234 (15)[g]	47 of 253 (19)	240 of 3959 (6)	12 of 152 (8)
Asymptomatic carriage	52 of 83 (63)	51 of 54 (94)	25 of 34 (74)	19 of 47 (40)	123 of 240 (51)	8 of 12 (75)
CDI	31 of 83 (37)	3 of 54 (6)	9 of 34 (26)	28 of 47 (60)	117 of 240 (49)	4 of 12 (25)
Persistence of carriage	68 of 83 (82) colonized on discharge[h]	—	44 of 71 (62) colonized on follow-up cultures	—	—	—

Abbreviation: ICU, intensive care unit.
[a] Includes toxigenic and nontoxigenic strains.
[b] Includes 406 subjects with initial culture within 72 hours of admission and 90 with initial culture greater than 72 hours after admission.
[c] Only toxigenic strains included based on real-time polymerase chain reaction and culture.
[d] Twenty-four of 44 (55%) toxigenic.
[e] Cytotoxin activity was detected in stools of 15 of 19 (79%) asymptomatic carriers and 3 of 4 with negative cytotoxin activity carried nontoxigenic strains.
[f] Seventy-five patients either developed CDI within 3 days of admission (n = 60) or were asymptomatically colonized on admission and subsequently developed CDI (n = 15).
[g] Nineteen of 34 (56%) toxigenic with 10 remaining asymptomatic and 9 developing CDI.
[h] Includes both asymptomatic carriers and patients with CDI.

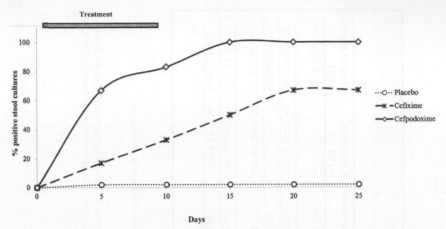

Fig. 1. Frequency of acquisition of *C difficile* stool colonization in healthy community-dwelling subjects receiving oral placebo, cefixime, or cefpodoxime. (*Adapted from* Chachaty E, Depitre C, Mario N, et al. Presence of *Clostridium difficile* and antibiotic and beta-lactamase activities in feces of volunteers treated with oral cefixime, oral cefpodoxime proxetil, or placebo. Antimicrob Agents Chemother 1992;36(9):2011; with permission. Copyright © 1992, American Society for Microbiology.)

ecology, the term colonization is typically indicated by the presence of a constant population of an invading bacterium over time, requiring that growth occurs at a rate equal to the rate of removal.[26] As discussed later, if the indigenous microbiota is intact, exposure to *C difficile* spores potentially results in transient carriage or pass-through with positive stool cultures without establishment of stable colonization. This phenomenon has been shown in animal models and also in healthy humans receiving nontoxigenic *C difficile* spores.[27]

The conclusions that can be drawn from epidemiologic studies evaluating carriage of *C difficile* are often limited because single cultures are collected or limited information is provided on the duration of carriage. From a practical point of view, recovery of *C difficile* from multiple specimens over a period of weeks is likely to indicate persistent colonization, whereas recovery of *C difficile* at a single time point could represent colonization or transient carriage or pass-through. The importance of this concept is shown by studies of community-dwelling adults. In 3 studies that included repeat testing, a minority of healthy adults with detectable *C difficile* in stool carried the same strain on follow-up testing (16%–33%).[21,22,24] Thus, detection of *C difficile* may have represented transient carriage rather than colonization in many subjects.

PATHOGENESIS OF INTESTINAL COLONIZATION

Fig. 2 provides an overview of the pathogenesis of *C difficile* colonization. Ingestion of spores may occur through exposure to a variety of sources, including food and water. In health care facilities, the hands of health care workers and contaminated environmental surfaces are common sources.

Gastric acid provides an important host defense by killing ingested pathogens.[28] However, the importance of gastric acid as a defense against *C difficile* is controversial. Many studies have shown an association between medications that inhibit stomach acid and CDI,[29] but not all studies have confirmed this association,[30] Moreover, the mechanism by which proton pump inhibitors may promote CDI is unclear

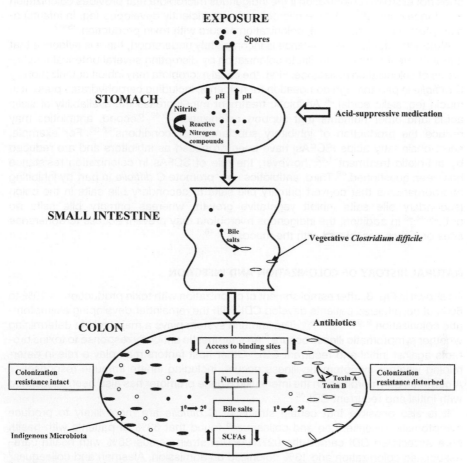

Fig. 2. Factors that facilitate intestinal colonization by *C difficile*. The left half of the circles represents the presence of normal acidity in the stomach and intact indigenous microbiota in the colon; the right half represents the effects of acid-suppressive medications and antibiotic therapy in the colon. In the stomach, acidic pH and reactive nitrogen compounds produced from acidified nitrite are not sufficient to kill spores (area of controversy). In the small intestine, spores germinate in response to bile salts and other germinants. In the colon, the indigenous microbiota provides colonization resistance through several potential mechanisms, including reducing access to binding sites or niches associated with the mucosa, competition for nutrients, and production of inhibitory substances such as secondary bile salts or short-chain fatty acids (SCFAs).

because acidic gastric contents do not kill spores and germination does not occur in gastric contents.[28,31] Under acidic conditions, salivary nitrites are converted to reactive nitrogen compounds that could potentially kill spores, but it is not clear that usual physiologic levels of nitrite are sufficient to provide sporicidal activity.[28,32] An alternative hypothesis is that proton pump inhibitor therapy may alter the intestinal microbiota.[33]

After spores pass through the stomach, they germinate in the small intestine in response to germinants, including bile salts.[34] In the colon, vegetative *C difficile* does not establish colonization if the indigenous microbiota that provides colonization resistance is intact.[35,36] If the microbiota is insufficiently developed (eg, in infants) or disrupted (eg, by antibiotics), colonization occurs with toxin production.[35–37]

Although colonization resistance is incompletely understood, there is evidence that antibiotic treatment may facilitate colonization by disrupting several potential mechanisms of colonization resistance. First, the cecal microbiota may inhibit colonization by *C difficile* in part through competition for nutrients, including carbohydrates present in mucin (eg, sialic acids).[38] Antibiotic treatment may increase the availability of sialic acids and other nutrients that support colonization.[39,40] Second, antibiotics may reduce the production of inhibitory substances or conditions.[26,36] For example, short-chain fatty acids (SCFAs) have been proposed as inhibitors and are reduced by antibiotic treatment[41,42]; however, the role of SCFAs in colonization resistance has been questioned.[43] Third, antibiotics may promote *C difficile* in part by inhibiting microorganisms that convert primary bile salts to secondary bile salts in the colon (secondary bile salts inhibit vegetative growth, whereas primary bile salts do not).[34,44,45] In addition, the indigenous microbiota may prevent access to adherence sites or niches associated with the mucosa.[26,46]

NATURAL HISTORY OF COLONIZATION AND INFECTION

As shown in **Fig. 3**, after establishment of colonization with toxin production, ~10% to 60% of hospitalized patients develop CDI, with the remainder developing asymptomatic colonization.[2–6,9–12,14,15,17] The immune system plays a major role in determining whether symptomatic illness occurs.[5] An anamnestic antibody response to toxins protects against initial and recurrent CDI.[5] Other host factors may play a role in determining whether symptomatic illness occurs, including innate immune responses.[47] A common polymorphism in the interleukin 8 gene promoter has also been associated with initial and recurrent CDI.[48]

It is also possible that certain strains of *C difficile* are more likely to produce symptomatic disease. Loo and colleagues[6] found that 63% of patients with health care–associated CDI carried the 027/NAP1/BI strain versus 36% with health care–associated colonization and 13% colonized on admission. Alasmari and colleagues[9] similarly found that ~25% of CDI cases were caused by the 027/NAP1/BI strain versus only 3% of asymptomatic carriers.

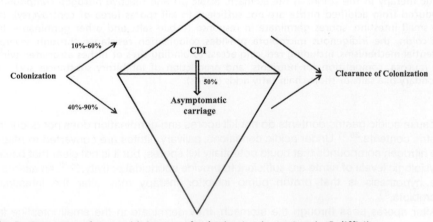

Fig. 3. Outcomes after establishment of colonization by toxigenic *C difficile*.

As shown in **Fig. 3**, patients with symptomatic CDI often continue to shed spores after symptom resolution.[8,49] **Fig. 4** provides more detail of the natural history of shedding of *C difficile* in patients with CDI based on 2 cohort studies.[8,50] At the time CDI testing is ordered and at diagnosis, all patients shed spores in stool and most had skin and environmental contamination. With effective treatment, shedding decreased markedly; at the end of treatment, 7%, 33%, and 15% had stool, skin, and environmental shedding, respectively. However, shedding increased after discontinuation of treatment, with 56% of patients with CDI persistently shedding spores for 1 month; the reduction in colonization after 1 month may coincide with recovery of colonization resistance.[51] In addition, asymptomatic carriage also precedes the onset of diarrhea, but the duration of carriage is likely to be short.[52]

Patients with previous CDI are an easily identified subset of asymptomatic carriers. In addition, they may make up a significant proportion of carriers. In point-prevalence surveys conducted in LTCF and hospital settings, patients with recent CDI accounted for 23% and 22% of all asymptomatic carriers, respectively.[14,18]

ANTIBIOTIC SELECTIVE PRESSURE AND COLONIZATION

Systemic antibiotic therapy may have a major impact on the natural history of colonization, the risk for shedding, and the strain types that are acquired.[53] Some important considerations regarding antibiotics and *C difficile* colonization include:

- Antibiotic-induced alteration of the intestinal microbiota may persist for days to weeks
- Antibiotics with inhibitory activity against *C difficile* may inhibit colonization during therapy but promote colonization if exposure occurs during the period of microbiota recovery (eg, piperacillin/tazobactam, oral vancomycin)
- Antibiotics lacking inhibitory activity against *C difficile* may promote colonization during and after therapy (eg, cephalosporins)

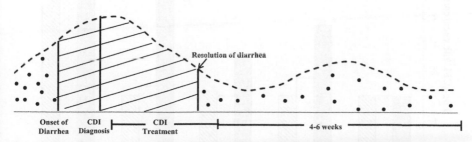

Fig. 4. Stool, skin, and environmental shedding of *C difficile* spores before, during, and after treatment of CDI. (*Adapted from* Sethi AK, Al-Nassir WN, Nerandzic MM, et al. Persistence of skin contamination and environmental shedding of *Clostridium difficile* during and after treatment of *C. difficile* infection. Infect Control Hosp Epidemiol 2010;31(1):23, with permission. © 2010 by Curtis J. Donskey; and Sunkesula VC, Kundrapu S, Jury LA, et al. Potential for transmission of spores by patients awaiting laboratory testing to confirm suspected *Clostridium difficile* infection. Infect Control Hosp Epidemiol 2013;34(3):307, with permission. © 2013 by Curtis J. Donskey.)

- As shown in **Fig. 5**, antibiotics may exert selective pressure favoring colonization by certain strains of *C difficile* (eg, fluoroquinolones may promote colonization by fluoroquinolone-resistant strains while inhibiting colonization with fluoroquinolone-susceptible strains)[35]
- Antibiotic therapy potentially converts individuals with low-level colonization into so-called supershedders with high-density stool colonization[41]

POTENTIAL FOR TRANSMISSION BY ASYMPTOMATIC CARRIERS

As shown in **Table 2**, several studies have shown that asymptomatic carriers often have skin and/or environmental shedding, albeit to a lesser degree than patients with CDI.[2,8,14,18,54–56] Asymptomatic carriers may have less frequent shedding than newly diagnosed patients with CDI because they have lower levels of *C difficile* in stool and they do not have diarrhea.[8,18] Increased density of organisms in stool has been associated with increased environmental and skin contamination.[8] Factors that reduce standards of hygiene (eg, altered mental status) may also contribute to skin contamination.

Although all asymptomatic carriers are typically grouped for analysis, subsets of carriers may present a particularly high or low risk of transmission. As shown in **Fig. 6**, the burden of colonization varied widely among asymptomatic carriers in an LTCF, and increased burden of colonization was associated with increased skin and/or environmental contamination.[54] There is a need for studies to clarify whether carriers with increased burden of colonization are more likely to transmit *C difficile*.

EVIDENCE THAT ASYMPTOMATIC CARRIERS CONTRIBUTE TO TRANSMISSION

Three studies that have included molecular typing have evaluated the role of adult asymptomatic carriers in transmission. On a medical-surgical ward, Clabots and

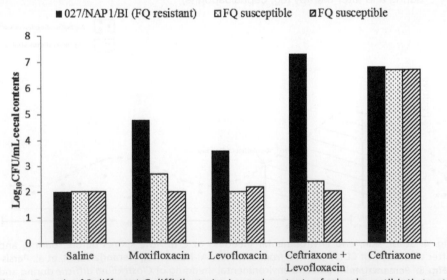

Fig. 5. Growth of 3 different *C difficile* strains in cecal contents of mice, by antibiotic treatment group. FQ, fluoroquinolone. (*Adapted from* Adams DA, Riggs MM, Donskey CJ. Effect of fluoroquinolone treatment on growth of and toxin production by epidemic and nonepidemic *Clostridium difficile* strains in the cecal contents of mice. Antimicrob Agents Chemother 2007;51(8):2674–8; with permission. Copyright © 2007 by Curtis J. Donskey.)

Table 2
Skin and environmental contamination in patients with CDI versus asymptomatic carriers

| | | No. Positive/No. Sampled (%) | | | |
| | | Patients with CDI | | Asymptomatic Carriers | |
Ref. #	Subjects	Skin	Environment	Skin	Environment
2	Medical ward	—	44 of 90 (49)	—	11 of 38 (29)
18	LTCF residents	14 of 18 (78)	14 of 18 (78)	21 of 35 (61)	20 of 35 (61)
14	Acute care	5 of 6 (83)	4 of 6 (67)	2 of 18 (11)	2 of 18 (11)
56	Oncology unit	—	19 of 97 (20)	—	5 of 74 (7)
54	LTCF residents	—	—	11 of 25 (44)	10 of 25 (40)
8	Acute care patients and LTCF residents[a]	—	—	15 of 26 (58)	13 of 26 (50)
55	Outpatients[a]	1 of 1 (100)	1 of 1 (100)	13 of 43 (30)	11 of 43 (26)

[a] All asymptomatic carriers were patients with prior CDI.

colleagues[3] found that 15 of 19 (79%) nosocomial acquisitions of *C difficile* were linked to asymptomatic carriers newly admitted to the study ward based on restriction enzyme analysis typing. Most of the carriers linked to transmission had been hospitalized within 30 days or were transferred from another ward (**Fig. 7**).

More recently, Curry and colleagues[11] used multilocus variable number of tandem repeats analysis genotyping to show that incident CDI cases in a tertiary care hospital were as frequently linked to asymptomatic carriers as to CDI cases (29% vs 30%,

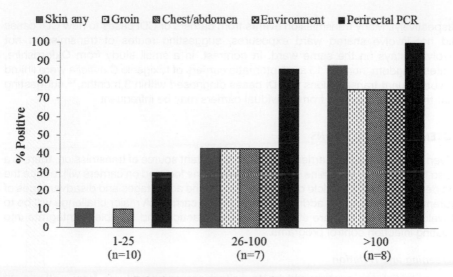

Colonies recovered per perirectal swab

Fig. 6. Percentages of positive perirectal polymerase chain reaction (PCR) results and skin and environmental cultures from LTCF residents with asymptomatic carriage of *C difficile*, stratified by the number of *C difficile* colonies recovered per swab. (*From* Donskey CJ, Sunkesula VC, Jencson AL, et al. Utility of a commercial PCR assay and a clinical prediction rule for detection of toxigenic *Clostridium difficile* in asymptomatic carriers. J Clin Microbiol 2014;52(1):317; with permission.)

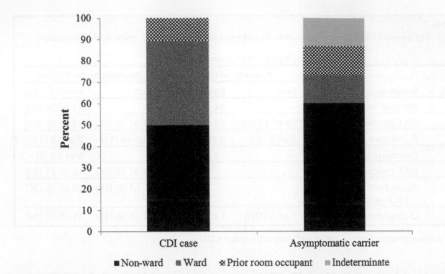

Fig. 7. Most likely transmission routes for incident CDI cases linked by multilocus variable number of tandem repeats analysis to CDI cases or asymptomatic carriers. Nonward, hospitalized concurrently or within 30 days without wards in common; ward, shared a common ward occupancy within 30 days; prior room occupant, incident CDI case occurred after placement in a room previously occupied by a CDI case or asymptomatic carrier. (*Data from* Curry SR, Muto CA, Schlackman JL, et al. Use of multilocus variable number of tandem repeats analysis genotyping to determine the role of asymptomatic carriers in *Clostridium difficile* transmission. Clin Infect Dis 2013;57(8):1095. Copyright © 2013, Oxford University Press.)

respectively). Many transmission events from carriers or CDI cases to new CDI cases did not involve shared ward exposures, suggesting routes of transmission not involving stays on the same ward. In contrast, in a small study from Oxfordshire, United Kingdom, none of 13 asymptomatic carriers of toxigenic *C difficile* were linked to subsequent transmissions to CDI cases diagnosed within 3 months,[12] suggesting that transmission events from individual carriers may be infrequent.

POTENTIAL INTERVENTIONS

Given the evidence that carriers may be an important source of transmission, there is a need for studies to determine whether interventions focused on carriers will reduce the incidence of CDI. This article discusses some of the advantages and disadvantages of potential interventions to address asymptomatic carriers. A major challenge will be to develop strategies that are effective but also practical and feasible to integrate into existing infection control programs.

Screening and Isolation

One potential approach would be to collect screening cultures from patients on admission and at intervals during their stay, and place asymptomatic carriers in contact precautions. Advantages of this approach include effectiveness in identifying most carriers and consistency with interventions used to prevent transmission of other pathogens. However, there are several disadvantages. Most microbiology laboratories are not adept at culturing *C difficile* and results are not available for several days. Although commercial polymerase chain reaction (PCR) assays could provide a rapid alternative to culture, the expense of screening would increase. In LTCF residents, a commercial PCR assay of perirectal swab specimens detected 68% of asymptomatic carriers of toxigenic *C difficile*, including 93% of those with skin and/or environmental contamination.[54] A clinical prediction rule including 2 factors (recent antibiotic use and previous CDI) provided a sensitive initial screen to identify a subset of high-risk patients for testing, thereby reducing the cost of screening.

Decolonization

Decolonization of intestinal carriage would address the major source of dissemination. However, in a randomized trial, oral vancomycin and metronidazole proved ineffective for decolonization of asymptomatic carriers.[57] As shown in **Fig. 8**, oral metronidazole did not suppress colonization, whereas oral vancomycin suppressed colonization during treatment, but subsequently was associated with more frequent colonization than controls. Metronidazole was not detectable in stool, consistent with other studies indicating that it does not achieve detectable levels in the absence of diarrhea.[58] The high frequency of colonization after vancomycin treatment may be caused by its disruption of the intestinal microbiota.[59] Fidaxomicin is a more selective agent that could potentially be used for decolonization.[60] However, no published data are available on the effectiveness of fidaxomicin for decolonization of carriers.

Focus on the Subset of Asymptomatic Carriers with Prior Clostridium difficile Infection

One potential strategy to address asymptomatic carriers would be to initially focus on patients with prior CDI. As noted previously, this subset of carriers is easily identified.

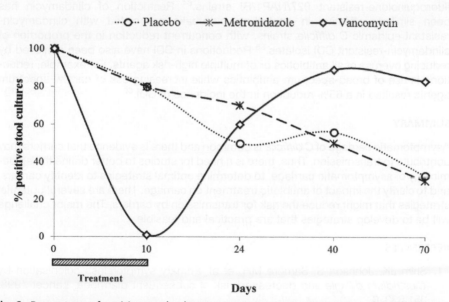

Fig. 8. Percentage of positive stool cultures among asymptomatic carriers of *C difficile* randomized to receive oral placebo, metronidazole, or vancomycin. (*Adapted from* Johnson S, Homann SR, Bettin KM, et al. Treatment of asymptomatic *Clostridium difficile* carriers (fecal excretors) with vancomycin or metronidazole. A randomized, placebo-controlled trial. Ann Intern Med 1992;117(4):299; with permission. Copyright © 1992, American College of Physicians.)

Interventions to address patients with recent CDI could include extending the duration of contact precautions or decolonization.

Skin and Environmental Disinfection

Disinfection of skin and environmental spore contamination could reduce the risk for transmission by asymptomatic carriers. Such strategies could be applied to carriers identified through screening or to all patients with no screening. However, alcohol hand hygiene products, chlorhexidine, and many environmental disinfectants do not kill spores.[61] Washing hands with soap and water and showering reduces spore contamination through mechanical removal.[61,62] Sporicidal skin disinfection products may be available in the future. For example, electrochemically activated saline solutions containing hypochlorous acid reduced levels of spores on skin when applied as a bed bath or hand hygiene solution.[63] Because asymptomatic carriers frequently contaminate environmental surfaces, use of sporicidal disinfectants routinely for all health care facility rooms could potentially reduce the risk for transmission without the requirement for screening for carriers.

Antimicrobial Stewardship Interventions

The simplest antimicrobial stewardship interventions involve formulary restriction of high-risk antibiotics. Third-generation cephalosporins have frequently been targeted because they have been associated with CDI and intestinal colonization with other pathogens.[53] Substitution of piperacillin/tazobactam, which has inhibitory activity against C difficile, for third-generation cephalosporins has been associated with reductions in CDI.[53] Restriction of fluoroquinolones has been associated not only with reductions in CDI but also with reductions in the proportion of infections caused by fluoroquinolone-resistant 027/NAP1/BI strains.[64] Restriction of clindamycin has been similarly effective in controlling outbreaks associated with clindamycin-resistant epidemic C difficile strains, with concurrent reduction in the proportion of clindamycin-resistant CDI isolates.[65] Reductions in CDI have also been achieved by reducing overuse of all antibiotics or of multiple high-risk agents. For example, reductions in use of broad-spectrum antibiotics while increasing use of narrow-spectrum agents resulted in a 65% reduction in the incidence of CDI.[66]

SUMMARY

Asymptomatic carriage of C difficile is common and there is evidence that carriers may contribute to transmission. Thus, there is a need for studies to better define the epidemiology of asymptomatic carriage, to determine optimal strategies to identify carriers, and to clarify the impact of antibiotic treatment on carriage. There are several potential strategies that might reduce the risk for transmission by carriers. The major challenge will be to develop strategies that are practical and feasible.

REFERENCES

1. Shim JK, Johnson S, Samore MH, et al. Primary symptomless colonisation by Clostridium difficile and decreased risk of subsequent diarrhoea. Lancet 1998; 351:633–6.
2. McFarland LV, Mulligan ME, Kwok RY, et al. Nosocomial acquisition of Clostridium difficile infection. N Engl J Med 1989;320:204–10.
3. Clabots CR, Johnson S, Olson MM, et al. Acquisition of Clostridium difficile by hospitalized patients: evidence for colonized new admissions as a source of infection. J Infect Dis 1992;166:561–7.

4. Samore MH, DeGirolami PC, Tlucko A, et al. *Clostridium difficile* colonization and diarrhea at a tertiary care hospital. Clin Infect Dis 1994;18:181–7.
5. Kyne L, Warny M, Qamar A, et al. Asymptomatic carriage of *Clostridium difficile* and serum levels of IgG antibody against toxin A. N Engl J Med 2000;342:390–7.
6. Loo VG, Bourgault AM, Poirier L, et al. Host and pathogen factors for *Clostridium difficile* infection and colonization. N Engl J Med 2011;365:1693–703.
7. Jinno S, Kundrapu S, Guerrero DM, et al. Potential for transmission of *Clostridium difficile* by asymptomatic acute care patients and long-term care facility residents with prior *C. difficile* infection. Infect Control Hosp Epidemiol 2012;33:638–9.
8. Sethi AK, Al-Nassir WN, Nerandzic MM, et al. Persistence of skin contamination and environmental shedding of *Clostridium difficile* during and after treatment of *C. difficile* infection. Infect Control Hosp Epidemiol 2010;31:21–7.
9. Alasmari F, Seiler SM, Hink T, et al. Prevalence and risk factors for asymptomatic *Clostridium difficile* carriage. Clin Infect Dis 2014;59:216–22.
10. Brazier JS, Fitzgerald TC, Hosein I, et al. Screening for carriage and nosocomial acquisition of *Clostridium difficile* by culture: a study of 284 admissions of elderly patients to six general hospitals in Wales. J Hosp Infect 1999;43:317–9.
11. Curry SR, Muto CA, Schlackman JL, et al. Use of multilocus variable number of tandem repeats analysis genotyping to determine the role of asymptomatic carriers in *Clostridium difficile* transmission. Clin Infect Dis 2013;57:1094–102.
12. Eyre DW, Griffiths D, Vaughan A, et al. Asymptomatic *Clostridium difficile* colonisation and onward transmission. PLoS One 2013;8:e78445.
13. Gerding DN, Olson MM, Peterson LR, et al. *Clostridium difficile*-associated diarrhea and colitis in adults. A prospective case-controlled epidemiologic study. Arch Intern Med 1986;146:95–100.
14. Guerrero DM, Becker JC, Eckstein EC, et al. Asymptomatic carriage of toxigenic *Clostridium difficile* by hospitalized patients. J Hosp Infect 2013;85:155–8.
15. Hung YP, Tsai PJ, Hung KH, et al. Impact of toxigenic *Clostridium difficile* colonization and infection among hospitalized adults at a district hospital in southern Taiwan. PLoS One 2012;7:e42415.
16. Johnson S, Clabots CR, Linn FV, et al. Nosocomial *Clostridium difficile* colonisation and disease. Lancet 1990;336:97–100.
17. Leekha S, Aronhalt KC, Sloan LM, et al. Asymptomatic *Clostridium difficile* colonization in a tertiary care hospital: admission prevalence and risk factors. Am J Infect Control 2013;41:390–3.
18. Riggs MM, Sethi AK, Zabarsky TF, et al. Asymptomatic carriers are a potential source for transmission of epidemic and nonepidemic *Clostridium difficile* strains among long-term care facility residents. Clin Infect Dis 2007;45:992–8.
19. Simor AE, Bradley SF, Strausbaugh LJ, et al. *Clostridium difficile* in long-term-care facilities for the elderly. Infect Control Hosp Epidemiol 2002;23:696–703.
20. Marciniak C, Chen D, Stein AC, et al. Prevalence of *Clostridium difficile* colonization at admission to rehabilitation. Arch Phys Med Rehabil 2006;87:1086–90.
21. Kato H, Kita H, Karasawa T, et al. Colonisation and transmission of *Clostridium difficile* in healthy individuals examined by PCR ribotyping and pulsed-field gel electrophoresis. J Med Microbiol 2001;50:720–7.
22. Ozaki E, Kato H, Kita H, et al. *Clostridium difficile* colonization in healthy adults: transient colonization and correlation with enterococcal colonization. J Med Microbiol 2004;53:167–72.
23. Rea MC, O'Sullivan O, Shanahan F, et al. *Clostridium difficile* carriage in elderly subjects and associated changes in the intestinal microbiota. J Clin Microbiol 2012;50:867–75.

24. Galdys AL, Curry SR, Harrison LH. Asymptomatic *Clostridium difficile* colonization as a reservoir for *Clostridium difficile* infection. Expert Rev Anti Infect Ther 2014;12:967–80.

25. Chachaty E, Depitre C, Mario N, et al. Presence of *Clostridium difficile* and antibiotic and beta-lactamase activities in feces of volunteers treated with oral cefixime, oral cefpodoxime proxetil, or placebo. Antimicrob Agents Chemother 1992;36:2009–13.

26. Freter R, Brickner H, Fekete J, et al. Survival and implantation of *Escherichia coli* in the intestinal tract. Infect Immun 1983;39:686–703.

27. Villano SA, Seiberling M, Tatarowicz W, et al. Evaluation of an oral suspension of VP20621, spores of nontoxigenic *Clostridium difficile* strain M3, in healthy subjects. Antimicrob Agents Chemother 2012;56:5224–9.

28. Rao A, Jump RL, Pultz NJ, et al. In vitro killing of nosocomial pathogens by acid and acidified nitrite. Antimicrob Agents Chemother 2006;50:3901–4.

29. Deshpande A, Pant C, Pasupuleti V, et al. Association between proton pump inhibitor therapy and *Clostridium difficile* infection in a meta-analysis. Clin Gastroenterol Hepatol 2012;10:225–33 [meta-analysis].

30. Naggie S, Miller BA, Zuzak KB, et al. A case-control study of community-associated *Clostridium difficile* infection: no role for proton pump inhibitors. Am J Med 2011;124(276):e271–7.

31. Nerandzic MM, Pultz MJ, Donskey CJ. Examination of potential mechanisms to explain the association between proton pump inhibitors and *Clostridium difficile* infection. Antimicrob Agents Chemother 2009;53:4133–7.

32. Cunningham R, Mustoe E, Spiller L, et al. Acidified nitrite: a host defence against colonization with *C. difficile* spores? J Hosp Infect 2014;86:155–7.

33. Vesper BJ, Jawdi A, Altman KW, et al. The effect of proton pump inhibitors on the human microbiota. Curr Drug Metab 2009;10:84–9.

34. Sorg JA, Sonenshein AL. Bile salts and glycine as cogerminants for *Clostridium difficile* spores. J Bacteriol 2008;190:2505–12.

35. Adams DA, Riggs MM, Donskey CJ. Effect of fluoroquinolone treatment on growth of and toxin production by epidemic and nonepidemic *Clostridium difficile* strains in the cecal contents of mice. Antimicrob Agents Chemother 2007;51:2674–8.

36. Pultz NJ, Stiefel U, Subramanyan S, et al. Mechanisms by which anaerobic microbiota inhibit the establishment in mice of intestinal colonization by vancomycin-resistant *Enterococcus*. J Infect Dis 2005;191:949–56.

37. Rousseau C, Poilane I, De Pontual L, et al. *Clostridium difficile* carriage in healthy infants in the community: a potential reservoir for pathogenic strains. Clin Infect Dis 2012;55:1209–15.

38. Wilson KH, Perini F. Role of competition for nutrients in suppression of *Clostridium difficile* by the colonic microflora. Infect Immun 1988;56:2610–4.

39. Ng KM, Ferreyra JA, Higginbottom SK, et al. Microbiota-liberated host sugars facilitate post-antibiotic expansion of enteric pathogens. Nature 2013;502:96–9.

40. Theriot CM, Koenigsknecht MJ, Carlson PE Jr, et al. Antibiotic-induced shifts in the mouse gut microbiome and metabolome increase susceptibility to *Clostridium difficile* infection. Nat Commun 2014;5:3114.

41. Lawley TD, Clare S, Walker AW, et al. Targeted restoration of the intestinal microbiota with a simple, defined bacteriotherapy resolves relapsing *Clostridium difficile* disease in mice. PLoS Pathog 2012;8:e1002995.

42. Rolfe RD. Role of volatile fatty acids in colonization resistance to *Clostridium difficile*. Infect Immun 1984;45:185–91.

43. Su WJ, Waechter MJ, Bourlioux P, et al. Role of volatile fatty acids in colonization resistance to *Clostridium difficile* in gnotobiotic mice. Infect Immun 1987;55: 1686–91.
44. Giel JL, Sorg JA, Sonenshein AL, et al. Metabolism of bile salts in mice influences spore germination in *Clostridium difficile*. PLoS One 2010;5:e8740.
45. Wilson KH. Efficiency of various bile salt preparations for stimulation of *Clostridium difficile* spore germination. J Clin Microbiol 1983;18:1017–9.
46. Banerjee P, Merkel GJ, Bhunia AK. *Lactobacillus delbrueckii* ssp. *bulgaricus* B-30892 can inhibit cytotoxic effects and adhesion of pathogenic *Clostridium difficile* to Caco-2 cells. Gut Pathog 2009;1:8.
47. Buffie CG, Pamer EG. Microbiota-mediated colonization resistance against intestinal pathogens. Nat Rev Immunol 2013;13:790–801.
48. Jiang ZD, DuPont HL, Garey K, et al. A common polymorphism in the interleukin 8 gene promoter is associated with *Clostridium difficile* diarrhea. Am J Gastroenterol 2006;101:1112–6.
49. Louie TJ, Cannon K, Byrne B, et al. Fidaxomicin preserves the intestinal microbiome during and after treatment of *Clostridium difficile* infection (CDI) and reduces both toxin reexpression and recurrence of CDI. Clin Infect Dis 2012; 55(Suppl 2):S132–42.
50. Sunkesula VC, Kundrapu S, Jury LA, et al. Potential for transmission of spores by patients awaiting laboratory testing to confirm suspected *Clostridium difficile* infection. Infect Control Hosp Epidemiol 2013;34:306–8.
51. Abujamel T, Cadnum JL, Jury LA, et al. Defining the vulnerable period for re-establishment of *Clostridium difficile* colonization after treatment of *C. difficile* infection with oral vancomycin or metronidazole. PLoS One 2013;8:e76269.
52. Centers for Disease Control and Prevention (CDC). Vital signs: preventing *Clostridium difficile* infections. MMWR Morb Mortal Wkly Rep 2012;61:157–62.
53. Owens RC Jr, Donskey CJ, Gaynes RP, et al. Antimicrobial-associated risk factors for *Clostridium difficile* infection. Clin Infect Dis 2008;46(Suppl 1):S19–31.
54. Donskey CJ, Sunkesula VC, Jencson AL, et al. Utility of a commercial PCR assay and a clinical prediction rule for detection of toxigenic *Clostridium difficile* in asymptomatic carriers. J Clin Microbiol 2014;52:315–8.
55. Jury LA, Sitzlar B, Kundrapu S, et al. Outpatient healthcare settings and transmission of *Clostridium difficile*. PLoS One 2013;8:e70175.
56. Kim KH, Fekety R, Batts DH, et al. Isolation of *Clostridium difficile* from the environment and contacts of patients with antibiotic-associated colitis. J Infect Dis 1981;143:42–50.
57. Johnson S, Homann SR, Bettin KM, et al. Treatment of asymptomatic *Clostridium difficile* carriers (fecal excretors) with vancomycin or metronidazole. A randomized, placebo-controlled trial. Ann Intern Med 1992;117:297–302.
58. Bolton RP, Culshaw MA. Faecal metronidazole concentrations during oral and intravenous therapy for antibiotic associated colitis due to *Clostridium difficile*. Gut 1986;27:1169–72.
59. Edlund C, Barkholt L, Olsson-Liljequist B, et al. Effect of vancomycin on intestinal flora of patients who previously received antimicrobial therapy. Clin Infect Dis 1997;25:729–32.
60. Louie TJ, Miller MA, Mullane KM, et al. Fidaxomicin versus vancomycin for *Clostridium difficile* infection. N Engl J Med 2011;364:422–31.
61. Kundrapu S, Sunkesula V, Jury I, et al. A randomized trial of soap and water hand wash versus alcohol hand rub for removal of *Clostridium difficile* spores from hands of patients. Infect Control Hosp Epidemiol 2014;35:204–6.

62. Jury LA, Guerrero DM, Burant CJ, et al. Effectiveness of routine patient bathing to decrease the burden of spores on the skin of patients with *Clostridium difficile* infection. Infect Control Hosp Epidemiol 2011;32:181–4.
63. Nerandzic MM, Rackaityte E, Jury LA, et al. Novel strategies for enhanced removal of persistent *Bacillus anthracis* surrogates and *Clostridium difficile* spores from skin. PLoS One 2013;8:e68706.
64. Kallen AJ, Thompson A, Ristaino P, et al. Complete restriction of fluoroquinolone use to control an outbreak of *Clostridium difficile* infection at a community hospital. Infect Control Hosp Epidemiol 2009;30:264–72.
65. Johnson S, Samore MH, Farrow KA, et al. Epidemics of diarrhea caused by a clindamycin-resistant strain of *Clostridium difficile* in four hospitals. N Engl J Med 1999;341:1645–51.
66. Fowler S, Webber A, Cooper BS, et al. Successful use of feedback to improve antibiotic prescribing and reduce *Clostridium difficile* infection: a controlled interrupted time series. J Antimicrob Chemother 2007;59:990–5.

Potential Sources of *Clostridium difficile* in Human Infection

Martijn P. Bauer, MD, PhD[a], Ed J. Kuijper, MD, PhD[b],*

KEYWORDS

- Animals • Food • Spores • Zoonosis • Transmission • Pigs
- Methicillin-resistant *Staphylococcus aureus* • PCR ribotype 078

KEY POINTS

- Zoonotic transmission of *Clostridium difficile* is possible.
- Spores of *C difficile* are ubiquitous.
- Asymptomatic colonization is a risk for transmission.
- Food-borne outbreaks of *C difficile* infection have not been observed.
- *C difficile* PCR ribotype 078 has crossed the species border.

The spore-forming anaerobic bacillus *Clostridium difficile* can be found worldwide in various environments, such as water, soil, and the digestive tracts of mammals. The spores are resilient and can survive high temperatures,[1] very dry and humid conditions, and various chemical attacks. Since the discovery of the etiologic agent, *C difficile* infection (CDI) in humans has been associated with health care facilities, where it occurs sporadically and in outbreaks. Therefore, health care facilities, especially hospitals, have been considered the most significant sources of *C difficile* acquisition. It was presumed that spores were spread by patients with diarrhea and, though to a lesser degree, asymptomatic carriers through fecal contamination of inanimate surfaces and the hands of health care workers, or through direct patient-to-patient contact. The presence of *C difficile* spores has been demonstrated on various surfaces in the hospital, especially in the vicinity of symptomatic patients.[2–4] The degree of environmental contamination in the hospital was found to correlate positively with transmission to patients and the hands of health care workers.[3,4] Furthermore, spores have been demonstrated in the air around patients with diarrhea.[5,6] Often during an

a Department of Infectious Diseases, Center for Infectious Diseases, Leiden University Medical Center, Albinusdreef 2, Leiden 2333 ZA, The Netherlands; b Department of Medical Microbiology, Center for Infectious Diseases, Leiden University Medical Center, Albinusdreef 2, Leiden 2333 ZA, The Netherlands
* Corresponding author.
E-mail address: E.J.Kuijper@lumc.nl

Infect Dis Clin N Am 29 (2015) 29–35
http://dx.doi.org/10.1016/j.idc.2014.11.010
0891-5520/15/$ – see front matter © 2015 Elsevier Inc. All rights reserved.

id.theclinics.com

outbreak no specific source can be identified, but specific inanimate sources that have been associated with CDI outbreaks include radiators[7] and rectal thermometers.[8] The most susceptible population, consisting of debilitated elderly patients with chronic comorbidity, could also serve as a reservoir in which C difficile could amplify.

However, the assumption that health care facilities are the most important source of C difficile acquisition has been challenged. In a study in the United Kingdom that used multilocus sequence typing, 75% of the isolates could not be linked to a case of CDI in the same hospital.[9] Links were established when patients spent time on the same ward, taking into account an infectious period of 8 weeks and an incubation period of 12 weeks. Potential weaknesses of the study were the assumptions regarding these infectious and incubation periods. Furthermore, patients could have come into contact with each other in places other than the ward, such as the waiting room of the radiology department. Most importantly, the importance of asymptomatic carriers in transmitting C difficile is unknown, and this study did not investigate asymptomatic carriage. Nonetheless, the study suggests that an important source of CDI is found outside of the hospital. A second study by the same group[10] used whole-genome sequencing to link CDI cases to other cases. When a difference of up to 2 single nucleotide variants between isolates was regarded as a genetic link, only 19% of CDI cases could be linked to a hospital contact. An additional 3% could be linked to other patients through potential community contact, defined as sharing the same general physician practice or living in the same postal-code district. The possibility exists that patients become colonized with C difficile outside of the hospital and then factors associated with the illness for which the patient is admitted (eg, changes in the intestinal microbiome because of the illness or antibiotic pressure) lead to symptomatic CDI in the hospital.

Additional evidence for the circulation of C difficile in the community comes from studies of community-onset CDI.[11–14] In these studies, many cases without an apparent link to health care were found, supported by molecular typing. Community-onset cases may go unnoticed because they can be self-limiting after the inciting antibiotic is stopped.[15]

If C difficile colonization is indeed acquired regularly outside of health care facilities, what could be the main reservoir and from what source might C difficile be acquired? CDI seldom occurs in outbreaks in the community, and therefore if humans are the main reservoir, C difficile is probably most often acquired from asymptomatic carriers. The recent finding that an emerging C difficile strain (polymerase chain reaction [PCR] ribotype 244) in Australia presents as community-onset CDI in more than 50% of cases illustrates how new types may develop in the community and subsequently spread to health care facilities, although a source of ribotype 244 in animals or food has not been found.[16] The prevalence of asymptomatic carriers in the community has rarely been investigated in an unbiased population. A study in healthy adults in Pennsylvania in 2012 and 2013 found a carriage rate of toxigenic C difficile of 6.6%.[17] Japanese studies from the beginning of the millennium found a carriage rate of approximately 10% in healthy adults.[18,19] Healthy infants have been implicated as an important reservoir, because they have been shown to have a high rate of colonization, mostly asymptomatic.[20] Contact with infants was found to be a risk factor for CDI among patients with community-onset diarrhea in the United Kingdom.[13] However, this observation was not confirmed in a large study performed in The Netherlands and Denmark.[21,22] The finding in some studies of a seasonal pattern for CDI, with a peak incidence in February, might also be consistent with transmission in the community.[23–25] One of these studies found that this peak was independent of the use of fluoroquinolones and macrolides.[24] The use of macrolides, which were presumably prescribed for respiratory infections, was higher in winter. CDI also seems to occur more often in cold climates, such as Canada, the Northern United States, and Northern Europe,[26] although this finding may be reflective of higher awareness. If climate influences CDI incidence, it seems plausible that this is caused by higher circulation in the community.

Could other important reservoirs exist in the community besides humans? As stated earlier, *C difficile* is present ubiquitously in water, both fresh and sea.[27,28] It has also been found in untreated and treated water from waste water treatment plants.[29,30] A Finnish study suggested that *C difficile* had been transmitted by drinking water contaminated with sewage, although the typing method used was too crude for strong conclusions to be made.[31] Furthermore, foods that come into contact with water could be sources of *C difficile* acquisition. Edible shellfish, known for their capacity to concentrate various pathogens from water through filter feeding, and other sea food and fish have been shown to contain *C difficile*.[32,33] An interesting recently completed study in Italy found that of 931 edible seashell samples, 18 (1.9%) were contaminated by *C difficile*. All mollusk farms that participated in the study performed routine quality control programs to survey fecal microbiological pollution. An unexpected inverse relationship between *C difficile* and *Salmonella* spp and *Escherichia coli* was found, suggesting that human feces are not the source of *C difficile* found in water (Troiano T, Harmanus C, Sanders IM, et al, unpublished data, 2014). Raw vegetables have also been shown to be contaminated by *C difficile* spores.[27,34–36]

Other potential reservoirs and sources for *C difficile* acquisition are animals and meat. CDI has been described in many animal species, including pigs, calves, horses, wild urban rats, poultry, ostriches, nonhuman primates, elephants, Kodiak bears, cats, and dogs.[21] In contrast to human studies, many studies in animals concentrate on the presence of the bacterium in healthy animals and the potential risk of spread to the environment and humans. A recently published Danish study of risk factors for CDI in the community revealed that contact with animals was a risk factor in a subgroup of patients.[22] The most studied animals are dogs, cats, horses, pigs and calves. An overlap exists between *C difficile* ribotypes isolated from animals and those from humans, although the hypervirulent *C difficile* ribotype 027 has only occasionally been found.[37–39] Investigations into the role of household pets as a possible reservoir of *C difficile* showed that colonization rates with mainly nonhuman types in healthy or diseased dogs and cats range from 1.4% to 21.0%.[39–41] Some *C difficile* ribotypes, such as 078 and 010, have been isolated from a few animal species only, suggesting a species-restricted occurrence. *C difficile* ribotype 078 was predominantly present in cattle and pigs,[42–44] and has already been proven to cross the species barrier to humans. In The Netherlands, an overlap between the location of pig farms and the occurrence of human *C difficile* ribotype 078 infections, which are increasing in prevalence, has been observed.[45,46] The fact that 078 is the predominant ribotype in piglets suggested a common source, which is likely to be the environment. Using whole-genome SNP analysis of *C difficile* ribotype 078 isolates collected from pigs (n = 19), farmers (n = 15), and hospitalized patients (n = 31), the authors recently demonstrated that farmers and pigs were colonized with identical or nearly identical *C difficile* clones.[47]

Data on colonization of calves and poultry in The Netherlands have been collected by Koene and colleagues,[40] who found that 6% of veal calves and 6% of poultry were positive for toxigenic ribotypes, which were clearly different from human-associated ribotypes. Contact with animals and pigs is currently being studied as a risk factor for colonization with *C difficile* in patients requiring hospitalization in a large prospective surveillance project in The Netherlands entitled "Livestock Farming and Neighboring Residents' Health, The VGO Study";[48] possible relationships among livestock farming, the environment, and the health of people living near farms are being studied. Livestock-associated methicillin-resistant *Staphylococcus aureus* and *C difficile* are both included.

Food products such as meat (processed), fish, and vegetables can also contain *C difficile*. Remarkably, studies conducted in Europe have persistently reported low prevalence rates (eg, ≤3% of meat samples), contrary to those conducted in the United States and Canada, where *C difficile* has been reported in up to 42% of meat samples,[49–55] although some of these rates may have been exaggerated because of laboratory contamination.[56] Meat has received the most attention, and information for other food products is limited. The source of contamination by *C difficile* in retail meat is unknown. It may involve fecal or environmental contamination of carcasses or contamination during processing by shedding handlers. Despite the presence of *C difficile* in cattle feces, spores of *C difficile* have not been reported in milk and milk products. However, the absolute counts of toxigenic *C difficile* in the environment and food are low. Despite the low numbers, the spore-forming nature of *C difficile* and the heat resistance of spores may facilitate food-borne transmission.

REFERENCES

1. Alfa MJ, Olson N, Buelow-Smith L, et al. Alkaline detergent combined with a routine ward bedpan washer disinfector cycle eradicates Clostridium difficile spores from the surface of plastic bedpans. Am J Infect Control 2013;41(4):381–3.
2. Fekety R, Kim KH, Brown D, et al. Epidemiology of antibiotic-associated colitis; isolation of Clostridium difficile from the hospital environment. Am J Med 1981; 70(4):906–8.
3. Samore MH, Venkataraman L, DeGirolami PC, et al. Clinical and molecular epidemiology of sporadic and clustered cases of nosocomial Clostridium difficile diarrhea. Am J Med 1996;100(1):32–40.
4. McFarland LV, Mulligan ME, Kwok RY, et al. Nosocomial acquisition of Clostridium difficile infection. N Engl J Med 1989;320(4):204–10.
5. Best EL, Fawley WN, Parnell P, et al. The potential for airborne dispersal of Clostridium difficile from symptomatic patients. Clin Infect Dis 2010;50(11):1450–7.
6. Roberts K, Smith CF, Snelling AM, et al. Aerial dissemination of Clostridium difficile spores. BMC Infect Dis 2008;8:7.
7. Teare EL, Corless D, Peacock A. Clostridium difficile in district general hospitals. J Hosp Infect 1998;39(3):241–2.
8. Brooks SE, Veal RO, Kramer M, et al. Reduction in the incidence of Clostridium difficile-associated diarrhea in an acute care hospital and a skilled nursing facility following replacement of electronic thermometers with single-use disposables. Infect Control Hosp Epidemiol 1992;13(2):98–103.
9. Walker AS, Eyre DW, Wyllie DH, et al. Characterisation of Clostridium difficile hospital ward-based transmission using extensive epidemiological data and molecular typing. PLoS Med 2012;9(2):e1001172.
10. Eyre DW, Cule ML, Wilson DJ, et al. Diverse sources of C. difficile infection identified on whole-genome sequencing. N Engl J Med 2013;369(13):1195–205.
11. Bauer MP, Veenendaal D, Verhoef L, et al. Clinical and microbiological characteristics of community-onset Clostridium difficile infection in The Netherlands. Clin Microbiol Infect 2009;15(12):1087–92.

12. Dial S, Delaney JA, Barkun AN, et al. Use of gastric acid-suppressive agents and the risk of community-acquired Clostridium difficile-associated disease. JAMA 2005;294(23):2989–95.
13. Wilcox MH, Mooney L, Bendall R, et al. A case-control study of community-associated Clostridium difficile infection. J Antimicrob Chemother 2008;62(2): 388–96.
14. Hensgens MP, Dekkers OM, Demeulemeester A, et al. Diarrhoea in general practice: when should a Clostridium difficile infection be considered? Results of a nested case-control study. Clin Microbiol Infect 2014. [Epub ahead of print].
15. Beaugerie L, Flahault A, Barbut F, et al. Antibiotic-associated diarrhoea and Clostridium difficile in the community. Aliment Pharmacol Ther 2003;17(7):905–12.
16. Lim SK, Stuart RL, Mackin KE, et al. Emergence of a ribotype 244 strain of Clostridium difficile associated with severe disease and related to the epidemic ribotype 027 strain. Clin Infect Dis 2014;58(12):1723–30.
17. Galdys AL, Nelson JS, Shutt KA, et al. Prevalence and duration of asymptomatic Clostridium difficile carriage among healthy subjects in Pittsburgh, Pennsylvania. J Clin Microbiol 2014;52(7):2406–9.
18. Kato H, Kita H, Karasawa T, et al. Colonisation and transmission of Clostridium difficile in healthy individuals examined by PCR ribotyping and pulsed-field gel electrophoresis. J Med Microbiol 2001;50(8):720–7.
19. Ozaki E, Kato H, Kita H, et al. Clostridium difficile colonization in healthy adults: transient colonization and correlation with enterococcal colonization. J Med Microbiol 2004;53(Pt 2):167–72.
20. Rousseau C, Lemee L, Le MA, et al. Prevalence and diversity of Clostridium difficile strains in infants. J Med Microbiol 2011;60(Pt 8):1112–8.
21. Hensgens MP, Keessen EC, Squire MM, et al. Clostridium difficile infection in the community: a zoonotic disease? Clin Microbiol Infect 2012;18(7):635–45.
22. Soes LM, Holt HM, Bottiger B, et al. Risk factors for Clostridium difficile infection in the community: a case-control study in patients in general practice, Denmark, 2009-2011. Epidemiol Infect 2014;142(7):1437–48.
23. Brown KA, Daneman N, Arora P, et al. The co-seasonality of pneumonia and influenza with Clostridium difficile infection in the United States, 1993-2008. Am J Epidemiol 2013;178(1):118–25.
24. Gilca R, Fortin E, Frenette C, et al. Seasonal variations in Clostridium difficile infections are associated with influenza and respiratory syncytial virus activity independently of antibiotic prescriptions: a time series analysis in Quebec, Canada. Antimicrob Agents Chemother 2012;56(2):639–46.
25. Reil M, Hensgens MP, Kuijper EJ, et al. Seasonality of Clostridium difficile infections in Southern Germany. Epidemiol Infect 2012;140(10):1787–93.
26. Bauer MP, Notermans DW, van Benthem BH, et al. Clostridium difficile infection in Europe: a hospital-based survey. Lancet 2011;377(9759):63–73.
27. al Saif N, Brazier JS. The distribution of Clostridium difficile in the environment of South Wales. J Med Microbiol 1996;45(2):133–7.
28. Zidaric V, Beigot S, Lapajne S, et al. The occurrence and high diversity of Clostridium difficile genotypes in rivers. Anaerobe 2010;16(4):371–5.
29. Romano V, Pasquale V, Krovacek K, et al. Toxigenic Clostridium difficile PCR ribotypes from wastewater treatment plants in southern Switzerland. Appl Environ Microbiol 2012;78(18):6643–6.
30. Xu C, Woese JS, Flemming C, et al. Fate of Clostridium difficile during wastewater treatment and incidence in Southern Ontario watersheds. J Appl Microbiol 2014; 117(3):891–904.

31. Kotila SM, Pitkanen T, Brazier J, et al. Clostridium difficile contamination of public tap water distribution system during a waterborne outbreak in Finland. Scand J Public Health 2013;41(5):541–5.
32. Pasquale V, Romano V, Rupnik M, et al. Occurrence of toxigenic Clostridium difficile in edible bivalve molluscs. Food Microbiol 2012;31(2):309–12.
33. Metcalf D, Avery BP, Janecko N, et al. Clostridium difficile in seafood and fish. Anaerobe 2011;17(2):85–6.
34. Eckert C, Burghoffer B, Barbut F. Contamination of ready-to-eat raw vegetables with Clostridium difficile in France. J Med Microbiol 2013;62(Pt 9):1435–8.
35. Metcalf DS, Costa MC, Dew WM, et al. Clostridium difficile in vegetables, Canada. Lett Appl Microbiol 2010;51(5):600–2.
36. Bakri MM, Brown DJ, Butcher JP, et al. Clostridium difficile in ready-to-eat salads, Scotland. Emerg Infect Dis 2009;15(5):817–8.
37. Lefebvre SL, Arroyo LG, Weese JS. Epidemic Clostridium difficile strain in hospital visitation dog. Emerg Infect Dis 2006;12(6):1036–7.
38. Songer JG, Trinh HT, Dial SM, et al. Equine colitis X associated with infection by Clostridium difficile NAP1/027. J Vet Diagn Invest 2009;21(3):377–80.
39. Wetterwik KJ, Trowald-Wigh G, Fernstrom LL, et al. Clostridium difficile in faeces from healthy dogs and dogs with diarrhea. Acta Vet Scand 2013;55:23.
40. Koene MG, Mevius D, Wagenaar JA, et al. Clostridium difficile in Dutch animals: their presence, characteristics and similarities with human isolates. Clin Microbiol Infect 2012;18(8):778–84.
41. Weese JS, Finley R, Reid-Smith RR, et al. Evaluation of Clostridium difficile in dogs and the household environment. Epidemiol Infect 2010;138(8):1100–4.
42. Rodriguez C, Avesani V, Van BJ, et al. Presence of Clostridium difficile in pigs and cattle intestinal contents and carcass contamination at the slaughterhouse in Belgium. Int J Food Microbiol 2013;166(2):256–62.
43. Schneeberg A, Neubauer H, Schmoock G, et al. Clostridium difficile genotypes in piglet populations in Germany. J Clin Microbiol 2013;51(11):3796–803.
44. Schneeberg A, Neubauer H, Schmoock G, et al. Presence of Clostridium difficile PCR ribotype clusters related to 033, 078 and 045 in diarrhoeic calves in Germany. J Med Microbiol 2013;62(Pt 8):1190–8.
45. Goorhuis A, Bakker D, Corver J, et al. Emergence of Clostridium difficile infection due to a new hypervirulent strain, polymerase chain reaction ribotype 078. Clin Infect Dis 2008;47(9):1162–70.
46. Keessen EC, Harmanus C, Dohmen W, et al. Clostridium difficile infection associated with pig farms. Emerg Infect Dis 2013;19(6):1032–4.
47. Knetsch CW, Connor T, Mutreja A, et al. Whole genome sequencing reveals potential spread of Clostridium difficile between humans and farm animals in the Netherlands, 2002 to 2011. Euro Surveill 2014;19(45). pii: 20954.
48. Maassen K. RIVM. Bilthoven, The Netherlands. Available at: http://vgo.sivz.nl/.
49. Harvey RB, Norman KN, Andrews K, et al. Clostridium difficile in retail meat and processing plants in Texas. J Vet Diagn Invest 2011;23(4):807–11.
50. Metcalf D, Reid-Smith RJ, Avery BP, et al. Prevalence of Clostridium difficile in retail pork. Can Vet J 2010;51(8):873–6.
51. Houser BA, Soehnlen MK, Wolfgang DR, et al. Prevalence of Clostridium difficile toxin genes in the feces of veal calves and incidence of ground veal contamination. Foodborne Pathog Dis 2012;9(1):32–6.
52. Weese JS, Avery BP, Rousseau J, et al. Detection and enumeration of Clostridium difficile spores in retail beef and pork. Appl Environ Microbiol 2009;75(15): 5009–11.

53. Rodriguez-Palacios A, Staempfli HR, Duffield T, et al. Clostridium difficile in retail ground meat, Canada. Emerg Infect Dis 2007;13(3):485–7.
54. Rodriguez-Palacios A, Reid-Smith RJ, Staempfli HR, et al. Possible seasonality of Clostridium difficile in retail meat, Canada. Emerg Infect Dis 2009;15(5):802–5.
55. Songer JG, Trinh HT, Killgore GE, et al. Clostridium difficile in retail meat products, USA, 2007. Emerg Infect Dis 2009;15(5):819–21.
56. Marsh JW, Tulenko MM, Shutt KA, et al. Multi-locus variable number tandem repeat analysis for investigation of the genetic association of Clostridium difficile isolates from food, food animals and humans. Anaerobe 2011;17(4):156–60.

The Epidemiology of *Clostridium difficile* Infection Inside and Outside Health Care Institutions

Dale N. Gerding, MD[a,b,*], Fernanda C. Lessa, MD, MPH[c]

KEYWORDS

- *Clostridium difficile* infection • Community associated • Health care associated
- Risk factors • Strain type

KEY POINTS

- *Clostridium difficile* has increased in incidence and severity, becoming the most common pathogen of health care–associated infections.
- The epidemiology of *C difficile* is shifting, with most patients having disease onset outside hospital settings.
- Most patients with onset of *C difficile* infection (CDI) in the community either had a recent inpatient or outpatient health care exposure, suggesting that *C difficile* continues to be largely a health care–associated pathogen.
- The molecular epidemiology of CDI is dynamic and other epidemic strains are likely to emerge.

Financial Disclosure: The authors have no financial relationships relevant to this article to disclose.

Conflict of Interest: Dr D.N. Gerding is a board member of Merck, Rebiotix, Summit, and Actelion, and consults for Sanofi Pasteur and Cubist, all of which perform research on potential *Clostridium difficile* products. Dr D.N. Gerding is a consultant for and has patents licensed to Shire, which makes vancomycin used to treat *C difficile* infection.

Disclaimer: The findings and conclusions in this article are those of the authors and do not necessarily represent the official position of the Centers for Disease Control and Prevention.

[a] Department of Medicine, Loyola University Chicago Stritch School of Medicine, 2160 S 1st Avenue, Maywood, IL 60153, USA; [b] Research Service, Edward Hines, Jr. Veterans Affairs Hospital, 5000 South Fifth Avenue, Building 1, Room 347, Hines, IL 60141, USA; [c] Division of Healthcare Quality Promotion, National Center for Emerging and Zoonotic Infectious Diseases, Centers for Disease Control and Prevention, 1600 Clifton Road, Atlanta, GA 30329, USA

* Corresponding author. Research Service, Edward Hines, Jr. Veterans Affairs Hospital, 5000 South Fifth Avenue, Building 1, Room 347, Hines, IL 60141.

E-mail address: dale.gerding2@va.gov

Infect Dis Clin N Am 29 (2015) 37–50

http://dx.doi.org/10.1016/j.idc.2014.11.004

0891-5520/15/$ – see front matter Published by Elsevier Inc.

id.theclinics.com

INTRODUCTION

Clostridium difficile is an unusual gastrointestinal bacterial infection highly associated with health care exposure and generally occurring only in subjects whose normal protective gut bacterial microbiota have been disrupted in some manner, usually by prior antimicrobial use. *C difficile* is ubiquitous in nature and able to survive for long periods in the environment through sporulation. Widespread presence of *C difficile* in animals (dogs, cats, pigs, calves, horses, sheep), particularly during their early development, and in common environmental sites such as surface water, drinking water, swimming pools, and soil has been shown.[1] In addition, low-level contamination of foods with *C difficile* spores has been found in beef, pork, turkey, shellfish, and a variety of ready-to-eat vegetables.[2–4] As a result of the widespread presence of *C difficile* spores and its long survival in the environment, it is highly likely that humans ingest *C difficile* frequently. However, because of limited antimicrobial exposure, most humans who ingest *C difficile* remain asymptomatic and uncolonized as a result of the colonization resistance of an intact gut microbiota.

HEALTH CARE–ASSOCIATED *CLOSTRIDIUM DIFFICILE* INFECTION

Although *C difficile* spores have widespread distribution in community sites, the initial clinical report of severe diarrhea and pseudomembranous colitis associated with clindamycin use came from a hospital setting in St Louis, Missouri, and precipitated the search for a causal agent eventually identified as *C difficile*.[5,6] Key factors in the occurrence of *C difficile* infection (CDI) in this hospital were the use of a new antibiotic, clindamycin, with an extensive antianaerobic bacterial spectrum coupled with the likely presence of *C difficile* in the hospital environment leading to exposure of highly susceptible patients to the organism. As early as 1979, it was shown that hospital environments are contaminated with *C difficile* spores.[7] Perhaps more importantly, *C difficile* contamination of the hands of hospital personnel and the environmental persistence of *C difficile* spores for up to 20 weeks was shown in 1981.[8] High rates of environmental spore contamination in hospitals are presumed to be the result of frequent CDI diarrheal episodes in hospitalized patients coupled with the resistance of spores to killing by environmental cleaners and disinfectants other than bleach.

Understanding of the epidemiology of CDI in health care settings was slow to emerge. It was not until 1986 that the first prospective case-control study of CDI was published, in which 87% of 149 CDI cases were found to be hospital associated.[9] *C difficile* was found in the stool of 21% of hospitalized case-matched control patients who did not have diarrhea, suggesting asymptomatic acquisition of *C difficile* in the hospital. CDI risk factors included receipt of clindamycin and receipt of multiple antibiotics for the treatment of infection within 14 days before CDI onset.[9] In a landmark article in 1989, McFarland and colleagues[10] used weekly rectal swab specimens to identify *C difficile* hospital acquisition in 21% of patients, most of whom (63%) were asymptomatic. The additional sophistication of molecular health care epidemiology was added by Johnson and colleagues,[11] who also used weekly rectal swab cultures plus restriction endonuclease analysis (REA) organism typing to document hospital acquisition of *C difficile* by 21% of patients, 82% of whom were asymptomatic. The use of REA typing identified 18 unique REA types of *C difficile* in these patients, but symptomatic CDI was caused only by 2 closely related REA types, B1 and B2, which were identified as causing a hospital outbreak of CDI at the time and suggesting the possibility of strain-related virulence variation in *C difficile*.[12]

Molecular strain typing was also used to show that admission to a hospital ward of asymptomatic patients carrying *C difficile* in their stool preceded acquisition of that specific strain of *C difficile* by other patients on that ward in 85% of acquisitions, indicating a possible role for asymptomatic colonized patients in transmission of *C difficile*.[13] Contrary to intuitive thinking based on methicillin-resistant *Staphylococcus aureus* and vancomycin-resistant enterococci epidemiology, asymptomatic patients colonized with *C difficile* have a significantly lower risk of developing CDI compared with uncolonized patients on the same hospital wards at the same time,[14] even though they may be a source of *C difficile* transmission to other patients. It is presumed that these asymptomatic colonized patients are protected from CDI either because they have developed antibodies against the *C difficile* toxins or they are colonized by harmless nontoxigenic strains of *C difficile* that lack toxin genes.[14,15]

The lack of a universally sensitive and reproducible typing system has slowed progress in the molecular epidemiology of CDI, but polymerase chain reaction (PCR) ribotyping, pulsed field gel electrophoresis (PFGE), multilocus variable-number tandem-repeat analysis, and REA have been the most frequent typing systems in use. Using REA typing, Belmares and colleagues[12] identified a total of 174 unique REA types over a 10-year period, two-thirds of which were sporadic and identified only in a single year. This finding compares with a tertiary referral hospital in which 55 unique REA types of *C difficile* were identified in a 1-year endemic period.[16] Belmares and colleagues[12] also identified large clusters of CDI cases (≥10 cases in consecutive months) caused by the same REA types, whereas smaller clusters (4–9 cases in consecutive months) were associated with a variety of other REA types. Taken together, these studies suggest that new *C difficile* strains are frequently introduced to hospitals from a large pool of strains, some of which result in hospital transmission to multiple patients, whereas most are sporadic and result in few or no transmissions. The source for these new strains is not well defined, but it is probably related to admissions and transfers of patients with active or recently resolved CDI and asymptomatically colonized patients.

Whole-genome sequencing (WGS) is the most sensitive and specific new method for molecular typing of *C difficile* isolates. In an early study using REA, 50% of second episodes of CDI (many of them multiple months after the previous episode) were caused by a new *C difficile* strain different from the original isolate (ie, reinfection)[17]; however, a more recent larger study of recurrence of CDI within 30 days after the end of treatment identified the same strain as the cause of recurrence in more than 80% of instances (ie, relapse).[18] The more sensitive WGS typing of these isolates confirmed the REA results indicating that relapses with the original strain are more common for recurrences within 30 days.[19] In a much larger epidemiologic study in the United Kingdom, WGS was used to type 1223 *C difficile* isolates using less than or equal to 2 single nucleotide variants to define identical strains and showed that only 38% of patients harboring identical strains had close contact with another symptomatic patient with CDI with the same strain. The investigators concluded that there must be diverse sources of *C difficile* other than symptomatic patients with CDI. The study was done during a nonoutbreak period of stable to declining endemic CDI rates in the United Kingdom and in the study hospital, did not include testing for asymptomatic colonized patients, and identified CDI cases using an insensitive enzyme immunoassay test for fecal toxin that could have resulted in failure to identify some CDI cases. Nonetheless, WGS elegantly documented the high number of different *C difficile* strains causing CDI and the lack of transmission that occurs with most of these strains as suggested in previous less sensitive typing studies.

Although large numbers of different *C difficile* strains have been found to cause CDI in hospitals endemically, when a health care–associated outbreak or epidemic occurs it is likely to be caused by a single or closely related strains that are being transmitted within the hospital.[12] Some of these epidemic strains have been reported in multiple hospitals that are often geographically distant from each other. For example, the REA J group caused outbreaks of CDI in multiple US hospitals in the 1990s and was also a leading outbreak strain in the United Kingdom, where it was shown by PCR ribotyping to be ribotype 001.[20,21] These J/001 strains were highly clindamycin resistant and increased CDI incidence was associated with prior clindamycin exposure in the patients infected with J/001 strains.[20] These epidemic strains result in outbreaks, but then diminish in frequency and are supplanted by new molecular types. Perhaps the most severe of these epidemic strains are the C difficile toxinotype III strains that first appeared in the United States and Canada at the turn of the twenty-first century. These strains produce a third or binary toxin, have a deletion and stop codon in the tcdC toxin regulator gene, and are characterized by PFGE as type NAP1, by REA as group BI, and by PCR as ribotype 027.[22,23] They are highly resistant to fluoroquinolone antibiotics and prior fluoroquinolone use has been identified as a risk factor.[23]

The health care epidemiology of CDI has changed markedly since the identification of BI/NAP1/027 C difficile outbreaks first in the United States and Canada, then rapidly spreading to the Europe. CDI caused by these strains is of particularly high severity, causing increased mortality and requiring increased use of colectomy to treat patients who are refractory to medical management.[22–25] In Montreal, health care–associated CDI (HA-CDI) incidence increased to as high as 22.5 CDI cases per 1000 discharges with a 30-day attributable mortality of 6.9%.[23] Subsequent elegant molecular studies have shown there were 2 distinct lineages of NAP1/BI/027 designated FQR1 and FQR2 that acquired both fluoroquinolone resistance mutations and a highly related conjugative transposon.[26] The strains subsequently spread throughout the world with the FQR1 lineage, which originated in and was widely disseminated in the United States, eventually spreading to Asia and Switzerland. The FQR2 lineage was found in multiple US sites and in Montreal in Canada and spread more widely than FQR1 to Europe. Rates of CDI overall, and specifically CDI caused by BI/NAP1/027, have decreased significantly in the United Kingdom but remain high in the United States, where 28.4% of 2057 recent C difficile isolates were NAP1.[25,27,28]

Recent reports suggest that the epidemiology of HA-CDI is changing. Rates of CDI in US hospitals have increased steadily since 1993 to more than 336,000 CDI hospitalizations in 2009, of which nearly one-third had CDI listed as the primary diagnosis.[29] In a 2011 prevalence survey across 183 US hospitals, C difficile was the most commonly reported pathogen (causing 12.1% of the health care–associated infections identified).[30] CDI continues to be a health care–associated infection, with 94% of all CDI being related to various precedent and concurrent health care exposures. However, some of these exposures are occurring in the outpatient setting, perhaps reflecting the increase in health care being delivered in the outpatient setting (Fig. 1).[31] In addition, 75% of CDIs now occur in nursing homes or in the community based on laboratory test identification, in contrast with the 87% of CDIs that were reported to be hospital onset in 1986.[9] Therefore, many patients are already admitted with CDI. Recent data from the US National Healthcare Safety Network showed that 52% of CDI patients already have CDI present at the time of hospital admission.[31] The overall rate of hospital-onset CDI in the 711 US acute-care hospitals in 2010 was 7.4 per 10,000 patient-days, with a median hospital rate of 5.4 per 10,000. Some patients were exposed to multiple health care settings; 20% of hospital-onset CDIs occurred in patients who were residents of a nursing home in the prior 12 weeks, and 67% of nursing home–onset CDI cases occurred in patients recently discharged from an acute-care hospital.[31]

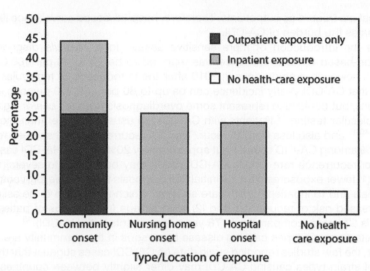

Fig. 1. Percentage of CDI cases (N = 10,342), by inpatient or outpatient status at time of stool collection and type/location of exposures (United States, Emerging Infections Program, 2010). (*From* Centers for Disease Control and Prevention. Vital signs: preventing *Clostridium difficile* infections. MMWR Morb Mortal Wkly Rep 2012;61:157–62.)

Nursing home or long-term-care residents seem to be at the highest risk of CDI within the first month of admission to the nursing home, when 52% to 69% of CDI cases in nursing homes are diagnosed, but overall rates of CDI per 10,000 patient-days are about 25% of those in acute-care hospitals in the same geographic area.[32,33] Among patients who developed CDI within the first month of admission to a nursing home, 68% were residents admitted for subacute care.[32] In a large study conducted across 33 nursing homes in New York, CDI resulted in hospitalization in 16% of the residents, 70% of whom had severe CDI.[33]

COMMUNITY-ASSOCIATED *CLOSTRIDIUM DIFFICILE* INFECTION

C difficile was thought to cause disease only in hospitalized and elderly patients until the beginning of the twenty-first century when reports of CDI in the community among young and previously healthy individuals in North America and Europe were published.[34–36] Since these initial reports, *C difficile* has been increasingly recognized outside health care settings.

The definition for community-associated CDI (CA-CDI) has differed among studies, especially before the publication of the interim surveillance definitions in 2007 by the Society for Healthcare Epidemiology of America, which defined CDI cases as community associated if patients had diarrhea onset in the community or within 48 hours after hospitalization and had not been discharged from a health care facility in the prior 12 weeks; otherwise CDI cases were defined as health care associated.[37] In addition to differences in surveillance definitions, some studies have also used different surveillance methods to identify CA-CDI. The proportion of total CDI cases that are reported to be CA-CDI ranges from 10% to 30% when using hospital-based surveillance and the recommended surveillance case definition,[38,39] but ranges from 30% to 50% when using population-based surveillance.[40–42] The lower proportion of CA-CDI in hospital-based studies can be explained by the report of Chitnis and colleagues,[43] which showed that approximately 25% of patients with CA-CDI are hospitalized;

thus, most are treated as outpatients. Therefore, hospital-based surveillance likely underestimates the burden of CA-CDI.

Before the introduction of more sensitive assays for *C difficile* diagnosis, the population-based CA-CDI incidence was reported to be 20 to 40 per 100,000 persons[39,44]; however, a study done in 2010 after the introduction of molecular assays showed that CA-CDI yearly incidence can be up to 80 per 100,000 persons in some US regions, but could also represent some overdiagnosis from the use of highly sensitive molecular testing.[42] Patients with CA-CDI are usually younger than those with HA-CDI,[45,46] and also less likely to recur. The CDI recurrence rate has been reported to be 10% among CA-CID cases[47] but approximately 20% among HA-CDI cases.[48,49] The lower recurrence rate among CA-CDI cases may be related to several factors, such as (1) fewer exposures after the initial CDI diagnosis to *C difficile*-provocative antimicrobials and to inpatient health care settings, which are known to be associated with increased risk of recurrence; and (2) younger age (median age of patients with CA-CDI is 53 years, compared with 78 years for patients with HA-CDI).[45]

The data on strain types causing disease in persons in the community are sparse. However, the few studies reporting strain data on CA-CDI cases suggest that the prevalence of strain types causing CA-CDI may differ slightly between countries. In the United States, the most common strain types in CA-CDI are PCR ribotype 027/ NAP1, which is the epidemic strain, ribotype 014/020 (primarily represents NAP4), and ribotype 016 (primarily represents NAP11).[43,45] In Europe, where decreases in the prevalence of ribotype 027/NAP1 are being observed,[28,29] the most prevalent strains causing CA-CDI are ribotypes 014/020, 106, and 015.[50,51] Ribotype 078 (or NAP 7/NAP8) is usually isolated from food and food animals, represents 2% to 7% of CA-CDI isolates in humans in both Europe and North America, and has the potential to cause severe disease.[43,45,52,53] Because the *C difficile* molecular epidemiology is both diverse and dynamic, as shown by Belmares and colleagues,[12] it is possible that other strains will emerge as important causes of CDI in the community. Recent reports from Australia and New Zealand[54,55] described the emergence of ribotype 244, toxinotype IX, causing severe CDI in the community and health care settings. Ribotype 244 produces binary toxin in addition to toxin A and toxin B but, unlike ribotype 027, it did not show high-level resistance to fluoroquinolones.

C difficile is a ubiquitous pathogen that may be found in the environment, food, and animals; therefore, the source of *C difficile* in CA-CDI is difficult to establish. A study by Chitnis and colleagues[43] involving telephone interviews of almost 1000 patients with CA-CDI showed that 82% of them had outpatient health care exposures such as doctor or dentist office visits, outpatient surgeries, or emergency department visits in the 12 weeks before the positive *C difficile* stool specimen. Outpatient settings can either be the place where antimicrobials, which disrupt the gut microbiota, are prescribed or a potential source of *C difficile* acquisition. In a study by Jury and colleagues,[56] toxigenic *C difficile* was isolated from several environmental surfaces in outpatient clinics and emergency departments with the providers' work areas and the patients' examination tables being the most frequently contaminated environmental sites. *C difficile* spores can survive for prolonged periods of time in the environment[57] and environmental disinfection in outpatient settings may be suboptimal because of high patient turnover.

In addition to outpatient settings, other potential sources of *C difficile* in the community have been described. Exposure to infants, who are known to have a high rate of *C difficile* colonization, and household members with active CDI have been reported to be associated with increased risk of CA-CDI.[44,58] *C difficile* has also been isolated from food and animals in several countries; however, its association with CDI in humans has not been shown. The prevalence of *C difficile* in retail meats has ranged substantially across studies; however, in most studies the prevalence is less than 7%.[59–61] The prevalence of *C difficile* in vegetables, including lettuce, potatoes, onions, carrot, radish, mushroom, and cucumber, is less understood. A study from France[2] reported that 2.9% of samples of ready-to-eat salad contained toxigenic *C difficile* strains, whereas a prevalence of 4.5% was reported in a similar study from Canada.[62] A recent study from Janezic and colleagues,[63] involving 112 *C difficile* isolates from 13 animal species in 12 different countries, showed a large variability of strains. Although ribotype 078 (or NAP 7) was the most prevalent, other ribotypes often found in humans, such as ribotype 014/020 and 002, were also common in animals across several countries. Some of the most prevalent strains among humans in the United States and part of Europe, including ribotype 027 (epidemic strain), ribotype 016, and ribotype 106,[27,43,53] were infrequently isolated from animals. Nevertheless, the partial overlap of strains between humans and animals increases the concern for potential zoonotic transmission, which needs to be further studied.

CLOSTRIDIUM DIFFICILE INFECTION IN CHILDREN

Reports of CDI in hospitalized children have increased substantially since 1997.[64,65] In the United States, rates of pediatric CDI-related hospitalizations went from 0.72 to 1.28 per 1000 hospitalizations from 1997 to 2006. Data from both hospital-based and population-based surveillance have shown that the highest CDI incidence is among children 1 to 4 years of age, with children 1 year old (ie, 12–23 months old) being the most affected; this is an age at which some asymptomatic *C difficile* colonization may still be present and may confound diagnostic testing, especially with the use of highly sensitive molecular methods such as PCR (**Fig. 2**).[65,66] According to population-based data, most (~70%) CDI in children is community associated and the hospitalization rate ranges from 11% to 25% depending on the age group.[67] CDI-related complications, including death, are rare in children. A prospective study among 82 hospitalized children with CDI found that toxic megacolon, gastrointestinal

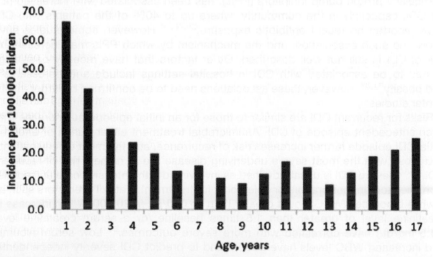

Fig. 2. Pediatric CDI crude incidence per 100,000 children by age, 2010 to 2011 (N = 944). (*From* Wendt JM, Cohen JA, Mu Y, et al. *Clostridium difficile* infection among children across diverse US geographic locations. Pediatrics 2014;133:653, with permission.)

perforation, pneumatosis intestinalis, and surgical intervention occurred in less than 2% of cases.[67] Although dedicated pediatric studies evaluating risk factors are limited in number, recent studies have suggested that children 1 year of age or older with co-morbid conditions such as cancer, solid organ transplant, gastrostomy, or jejunostomy are at increased risk for CDI.[68,69]

Infants less than 1 year of age have a high rate ($\sim$70%) of C difficile colonization by toxigenic and nontoxigenic strains[70,71] and are usually excluded from pediatric studies because it is difficult to differentiate colonization from infection in this age group. Asymptomatic colonization decreases rapidly during the second and third years and, by the time children reach 3 years of age, the rate of C difficile asymptomatic carriage is 0% to 3%, which is similar to that of adults.[72] Some experts have speculated that infants do not develop clinical illness even when colonized with toxigenic strains because of the absence of mature intestinal receptors for C difficile toxins as shown in rabbits, but this hypothesis has yet to be proved in humans.[71,73] The current recommendations advise against testing of C difficile in infants less than 1 year of age in the United States and less than 2 years of age in the United Kingdom. However, further studies are needed to determine how often C difficile causes disease in non-newborn children less than 2 years of age.

CLOSTRIDIUM DIFFICILE INFECTION RISK FACTORS

Risk factors for CDI, for recurrent CDI, for CDI severity, and for CDI caused by the epidemic NAP1/BI/027 strain are summarized in **Box 1**. The risk for developing CDI is dominated by prior antimicrobial exposure and increases with the duration and number of antimicrobials received.[74] Risk is highest during therapy and for the first month after antimicrobial therapy, and decreases between 1 and 3 months after antibiotic use.[75] Highest risk for CDI occurs with clindamycin, fluoroquinolones, and second-generation and higher cephalosporins.[76] Other important CDI risk factors are advanced patient age, immunosuppression, prior hospitalization, and increased severity of underlying illness.[77] The use of acid-suppressive agents, particularly proton pump inhibitors (PPIs), has been associated with increased risk for CDI, especially in the community, where up to 40% of the patients with CDI have reported no recent antibiotic exposure.[36,78,79] However, some studies have shown no such association, and the mechanism by which PPIs may increase the risk of CDI is still not well described. Other factors that have recently been suggested to be associated with CDI in hospital settings include antidepressants[80] and obesity[81,82]; however, these associations need to be confirmed by larger, multi-center studies.

Risks for recurrent CDI are similar to those for an initial episode but increase with each antecedent episode of CDI. Antimicrobial treatment either during or after the initial CDI episode further increases risk of recurrence, and the most elderly patients and those with the most severe underlying disease are at highest risk of recurrent CDI.[83,84] Severe CDI is usually defined as involving death, intensive care unit admission, megacolon, perforation, or colectomy for treatment. Patient predictors such as a white blood cell (WBC) count greater than 15,000/μL or 20,000/μL, an increase in creatinine level of greater than 1.5 times baseline (or a serum creatinine level $\geq$1.5 mg/dL) have correlated with more severe outcomes.[85] Low serum albumin and increased WBC levels have been found to predict CDI severity independently of infecting strain type, but higher 14-day mortality has been observed with infection caused by 2 strains of C difficile, NAP7-8-9/BK/078 and NAP1/BI/027, as well as with the presence of increased WBC and C-reactive protein levels, and low serum

---

Box 1

Risks for development of primary CDI, recurrent CDI, severe CDI, and CDI caused by the epidemic BI/NAP1/027 strain of *C difficile*

Risk factors for development of primary CDI

- Antibiotic exposure
- Increased patient age
- Prior hospitalization
- Severity of underlying illness
- Proton pump inhibitors and H2 blockers
- Abdominal surgery
- Nasogastric tube
- Long duration of hospitalization
- Long-term care residency

Risk factors for development of recurrent CDI

- Any prior episodes of CDI
- Additional antibiotic use
- Advanced age
- Prolonged or recent stay in health care facility
- High severity of Horn Index for underlying illness
- Proton pump inhibitor use
- Infection with NAP1/BI/027 strain type
- Absence of an antitoxin A antibody response

Risk factors for development of severe CDI

- White blood cell count greater than 15,000/μL
- Serum creatinine level greater than 1.5 × baseline
- Low serum albumin level
- Increased C-reactive protein level
- Infection with NAP7-8-9/BK/078 and NAP1/BI/027 *C difficile* strains

Risk factors for development of CDI caused by BI/NAP1/027 C difficile

- Age greater than 65 years
- Fluoroquinolone antibiotic exposure

---

albumin level.[52] Several studies have shown the association between infection with NAP1/BI/027 strains and increased disease severity,[25,52] but this has not been a universal finding.[86] A meta-analysis and strain risk comparisons have identified fluoroquinolone exposure and age more than 65 years as risks for CDI caused by NAP1/BI/027.[87]

SUMMARY

The epidemiology of *C difficile* inside and outside health care settings has changed markedly over the last decade since the emergence of the BI/NAP1/07 strain. *C difficile* is now the most common health care–associated pathogen and is no longer restricted to health care settings. It has emerged as an important cause of diarrhea in the community, with an annual incidence of CA-CDI as high as 80 per 100,000 persons in some regions. Although *C difficile* is a ubiquitous pathogen that has been isolated from the environment, food, and animals, the mechanisms of *C difficile* acquisition in the community are still poorly understood. However, the high proportion of CA-CDI cases with exposure to outpatient health care settings suggests that *C difficile* largely remains a health care–associated pathogen. Patients exposed to antimicrobials are at high risk of developing disease both in the community and in health care settings. However, other drugs, such as acid-suppressive agents, have been associated with increased risk of CDI, especially in the community. Because the molecular epidemiology of *C difficile* is both diverse (with numerous molecular types causing CDI) and dynamic (with changing dominance of strains), it is likely that new strains will emerge as epidemic strains and that understanding of the epidemiology of this microorganism will continue to evolve.

REFERENCES

1. al Saif N, Brazier JS. The distribution of *Clostridium difficile* in the environment of South Wales. J Med Microbiol 1996;45:133–7.
2. Eckert C, Burghoffer B, Barbut F. Contamination of ready-to-eat raw vegetables with *Clostridium difficile* in France. J Med Microbiol 2013;62(Pt 9):1435–8.
3. Pasquale V, Romano V, Rupnik M, et al. Occurrence of toxigenic *Clostridium difficile* in edible bivalve molluscs. Food Microbiol 2012;31:309–12.
4. Curry SR, Marsh JW, Schlackman JL, et al. Prevalence of *Clostridium difficile* in uncooked ground meat products from Pittsburgh, Pennsylvania. Appl Environ Microbiol 2012;78(12):4183–6.
5. Tedesco FJ, Barton RW, Alpers DH. Clindamycin-associated colitis. A prospective study. Ann Intern Med 1974;81:429–33.
6. Bartlett JG, Chang TW, Gurwith M, et al. Antibiotic-associated pseudomembranous colitis due to toxin-producing clostridia. N Engl J Med 1978;298:531–4.
7. Mulligan ME, Rolfe RD, Finegold SM, et al. Contamination of a hospital environment by *Clostridium difficile*. Curr Microbiol 1979;3:173–5.
8. Kim KH, Fekety R, Batts DH, et al. Isolation of *Clostridium difficile* from the environment and contacts of patients with antibiotic-associated colitis. J Infect Dis 1981;143(1):42–50.
9. Gerding DN, Olson MM, Peterson LR, et al. *Clostridium difficile*-associated diarrhea and colitis in adults. A prospective case-controlled epidemiologic study. Arch Intern Med 1986;146:95–100.
10. McFarland LV, Mulligan ME, Kwok RY, et al. Nosocomial acquisition of *Clostridium difficile* infection. N Engl J Med 1989;320(4):204–10.
11. Johnson S, Clabots CR, Linn FV, et al. Nosocomial *Clostridium difficile* colonisation and disease. Lancet 1990;336(8707):97–100.
12. Belmares J, Johnson S, Parada JP, et al. MD. Molecular epidemiology of *Clostridium difficile* over 10 years in one tertiary care hospital. Clin Infect Dis 2009;49:1141–7.
13. Clabots CR, Johnson S, Olson MM, et al. Acquisition of *Clostridium difficile* by hospitalized patients: evidence for colonized new admissions as a source of infection. J Infect Dis 1992;166(3):561–7.
14. Shim JK, Johnson S, Samore MH, et al. Primary symptomless colonisation by *Clostridium difficile* and decreased risk of subsequent diarrhoea. Lancet 1998;351(9103):633–6.

15. Kyne L, Warny M, Qamar A, et al. Asymptomatic carriage of *Clostridium difficile* and serum levels of IgG antibody against toxin A. N Engl J Med 2000;342(6):390–7.
16. Samore MH, Bettin KM, DeGirolami PC, et al. Wide diversity of *Clostridium difficile* types at a tertiary referral hospital. J Infect Dis 1994;170:615–21.
17. Johnson S, Adelmann A, Clabots CR, et al. Recurrences of *Clostridium difficile* diarrhea not caused by the original infecting organism. J Infect Dis 1989;159: 340–3.
18. Figueroa I, Johnson S, Sambol SP, et al. Relapse versus reinfection: recurrent *Clostridium difficile* infection following treatment with fidaxomicin or vancomycin. Clin Infect Dis 2012;55(Suppl 2):S104–9.
19. Eyre DW, Babakhani F, Griffiths D, et al. Whole-genome sequencing demonstrates that fidaxomicin is superior to vancomycin for preventing reinfection and relapse of infection with *Clostridium difficile*. J Infect Dis 2014;209:1446–51.
20. Johnson S, Samore MH, Farrow KA, et al. Epidemics of diarrhea caused by a clindamycin-resistant strain of *Clostridium difficile* in four hospitals. N Engl J Med 1999;341:1645–51.
21. Verity P, Wilcox MH, Fawley W, et al. Prospective evaluation of environmental contamination by *Clostridium difficile* in isolation side rooms. J Hosp Infect 2001;49:204–9.
22. McDonald LC, Killgore GE, Thompson A, et al. An epidemic, toxin gene-variant strain of *Clostridium difficile*. N Engl J Med 2005;353:2433–41.
23. Loo VG, Poirier L, Miller MA, et al. A predominantly clonal multi-institutional outbreak of *Clostridium difficile*-associated diarrhea with high morbidity and mortality. N Engl J Med 2005;353:2442–9.
24. Dallal RM, Harbrecht BG, Boujoukas AJ, et al. Fulminant *Clostridium difficile*: an underappreciated and increasing cause of death and complications. Ann Surg 2002;235:363–72.
25. See I, Mu Y, Cohen J, et al. NAP1 strain type predicts outcomes from *Clostridium difficile* infection. Clin Infect Dis 2014;58:1394–400.
26. He M, Miyajima F, Roberts P, et al. Emergence and global spread of epidemic healthcare-associated *Clostridium difficile*. Nat Genet 2013;45:109–13.
27. Wilcox MH, Shetty N, Fawley WN, et al. Changing epidemiology of *Clostridium difficile* infection following the introduction of a national ribotyping-based surveillance scheme in England. Clin Infect Dis 2012;55:1056–63.
28. Health Protection Agency (United Kingdom). Quarterly epidemiological commentary: mandatory MRSA & MSSA bacteraemia, and *Clostridium difficile* infection data (up to July – September 2011). London: Health Protection Agency; 2011. Available at: http://www.hpa.org.uk/webc/hpawebfile/hpaweb_c/1284473407318.
29. Lucado J, Gould C, Elixhauser A. *Clostridium difficile* infections (CDI) in hospital stays, 2009. HCUP statistical brief no. 124. Rockville (MD): US Department of Health and Human Services, Agency for Healthcare Research and Quality; 2011. Available at: http://www.hcup-us.ahrq.gov/reports/statbriefs/sb124.pdf.
30. Magill SS, Edwards JR, Bamberg W, et al. Multistate point-prevalence survey of health care-associated infections. N Engl J Med 2014;370(13):1198–208.
31. Centers for Disease Control and Prevention. Vital signs: preventing *Clostridium difficile* infections. MMWR Morb Mortal Wkly Rep 2012;61:157–62.
32. Mylotte JM, Russell S, Sackett B, et al. Surveillance for *Clostridium difficile* infection in nursing homes. J Am Geriatr Soc 2013;61(1):122–5.
33. Pawar D, Tsay R, Nelson DS, et al. Burden of *Clostridium difficile* infection in long-term care facilities in Monroe County, New York. Infect Control Hosp Epidemiol 2012;33:1107–12.

34. Centers for Disease Control and Prevention (CDC). Severe *Clostridium difficile*-associated disease in populations previously at low risk—four states, 2005. MMWR Morb Mortal Wkly Rep 2005;54:1201–5.
35. Norén T, Akerlund T, Bäck E, et al. Molecular epidemiology of hospital-associated and community-acquired *Clostridium difficile* infection in a Swedish county. J Clin Microbiol 2004;42:3635–43.
36. Dial S, Delaney JA, Barkun AN, et al. Use of gastric acid-suppressive agents and the risk of community-acquired *Clostridium difficile*-associated disease. JAMA 2005;294:2989–95.
37. McDonald LC, Coignard B, Dubberke E, et al. Ad Hoc *Clostridium difficile* Surveillance Working Group. Recommendations for surveillance of *Clostridium difficile*-associated disease. Infect Control Hosp Epidemiol 2007;28:140–5.
38. Shears P, Prtak L, Duckworth R. Hospital-based epidemiology: a strategy for 'dealing with *Clostridium difficile*'. J Hosp Infect 2010;74:319–25.
39. Kutty PK, Woods CW, Sena AC, et al. Risk factors for and estimated incidence of community-associated *Clostridium difficile* infection, North Carolina, USA. Emerg Infect Dis 2010;16:197–204.
40. Lambert PJ, Dyck M, Thompson LH, et al. Population-based surveillance of *Clostridium difficile* infection in Manitoba, Canada, by using interim surveillance definitions. Infect Control Hosp Epidemiol 2009;30:945–51.
41. Khanna S, Pardi DS, Aronson SL, et al. The epidemiology of community-acquired *Clostridium difficile* infection: a population-based study. Am J Gastroenterol 2012;107:89–95.
42. Lessa FC, Mu Y, Winston L, et al. Determinants of *Clostridium difficile* infection incidence across diverse US geographic locations. Pediatrics 2014;133(4):651–8. http://dx.doi.org/10.1093/ofid/ofu048.
43. Chitnis AS, Holzbauer SM, Belflower RM, et al. Epidemiology of community-associated *Clostridium difficile* infection, 2009 through 2011. JAMA Intern Med 2013;173:1359–67.
44. Wilcox MH, Mooney L, Bendall R, et al. A case-control study of community-associated *Clostridium difficile* infection. J Antimicrob Chemother 2008;62:388–96.
45. Dumyati G, Stevens V, Hannett GE, et al. Community-associated *Clostridium difficile* infections, Monroe County, New York, USA. Emerg Infect Dis 2012;18:392–400.
46. Hensgens MP, Keessen EC, Squire MM, et al. European Society of Clinical Microbiology and Infectious Diseases study group for *Clostridium difficile* (ESGCD). *Clostridium difficile* infection in the community: a zoonotic disease? Clin Microbiol Infect 2012;18:635–45.
47. Lessa FC. Community-associated *Clostridium difficile* infection: how real is it? Anaerobe 2013;24:121–3.
48. Eyre DW, Walker AS, Wyllie D, et al. Predictors of first recurrence of *Clostridium difficile* infection: implications for initial management. Clin Infect Dis 2012;55(Suppl 2):S77–87.
49. Lowy I, Molrine DC, Leav BA, et al. Treatment with monoclonal antibodies against *Clostridium difficile* toxins. N Engl J Med 2010;362:197–205.
50. Bauer MP, Notermans DW, van Benthem BH, et al. *Clostridium difficile* infection in Europe: a hospital-based survey. Lancet 2011;377:63–73.
51. Hensgens MP, Goorhuis A, Notermans DW, et al. Decrease of hypervirulent *Clostridium difficile* PCR ribotype 027 in the Netherlands. Euro Surveill 2009;14(45):pii (19402). Available at: http://www.eurosurveillance.org/ViewArticle.aspx?ArticleId=19402.

52. Walker AS, Eyre DW, Wyllie DH, et al. Relationship between bacterial strain type, host biomarkers, and mortality in *Clostridium difficile* infection. Clin Infect Dis 2013;56:1589–600.
53. Søes LM, Holt HM, Böttiger B, et al. The incidence and clinical symptomatology of *Clostridium difficile* infections in a community setting in a cohort of Danish patients attending general practice. Eur J Clin Microbiol Infect Dis 2014;33:957–67.
54. De Almeida MN, Heffernan H, Dervan A, et al. Severe *Clostridium difficile* infection in New Zealand associated with an emerging strain, PCR-ribotype 244. N Z Med J 2013;126:9–14.
55. Lim SK, Stuart RL, Mackin KE, et al. Emergence of a ribotype 244 strain of *Clostridium difficile* associated with severe disease and related to the epidemic ribotype 027 strain. Clin Infect Dis 2014;58:1723–30.
56. Jury LA, Sitzlar B, Kundrapu S, et al. Outpatient healthcare settings and transmission of *Clostridium difficile*. PLoS One 2013;8:e70175.
57. Bartlett JG. Historical perspectives on studies of *Clostridium difficile* and *C. difficile* infection. Clin Infect Dis 2008;46(Suppl 1):S4–11.
58. Pépin J, Gonzales M, Valiquette L. Risk of secondary cases of *Clostridium difficile* infection among household contacts of index cases. J Infect 2012;64:387–90.
59. Limbago B, Thompson AD, Greene SA, et al. Development of a consensus method for culture of *Clostridium difficile* from meat and its use in a survey of U.S. retail meats. Food Microbiol 2012;32:448–51.
60. Rodriguez-Palacios A, Reid-Smith RJ, Staempfli HR, et al. Possible seasonality of *Clostridium difficile* in retail meat, Canada. Emerg Infect Dis 2009;15(5):802–5.
61. Hoover DG, Rodriguez-Palacios A. Transmission of *Clostridium difficile* in foods. Infect Dis Clin North Am 2013;27:675–85.
62. Metcalf DS, Costa MC, Dew WM, et al. *Clostridium difficile* in vegetables, Canada. Lett Appl Microbiol 2010;51:600–2.
63. Janezic S, Zidaric V, Pardon B, et al. International *Clostridium difficile* animal strain collection and large diversity of animal associated strains. BMC Microbiol 2014;14:173.
64. Kim J, Smathers SA, Prasad P, et al. Epidemiological features of *Clostridium difficile*-associated disease among inpatients at children's hospitals in the United States, 2001-2006. Pediatrics 2008;122:1266–70.
65. Zilberberg MD, Tillotson GS, McDonald C. *Clostridium difficile* infections among hospitalized children, United States, 1997-2006. Emerg Infect Dis 2010;16:604–9.
66. Wendt JM, Cohen JA, Mu Y, et al. *Clostridium difficile* infection among children across diverse US geographic locations. Pediatrics 2014;133:651–8.
67. Kim J, Shaklee JF, Smathers S, et al. Risk factors and outcomes associated with severe *Clostridium difficile* infection in children. Pediatr Infect Dis J 2012;31:134–8.
68. Sandora TJ, Fung M, Flaherty K, et al. Epidemiology and risk factors for *Clostridium difficile* infection in children. Pediatr Infect Dis J 2011;30:580–4.
69. Tai E, Richardson LC, Townsend J, et al. *Clostridium difficile* infection among children with cancer. Pediatr Infect Dis J 2011;30:610–2.
70. Tullus K, Aronsson B, Marcus S, et al. Intestinal colonization with *Clostridium difficile* in infants up to 18 months of age. Eur J Clin Microbiol Infect Dis 1989;8:390–3.
71. Rousseau C, Poilane I, De Pontual L, et al. *Clostridium difficile* carriage in healthy infants in the community: a potential reservoir for pathogenic strains. Clin Infect Dis 2012;55:1209–15.
72. Jangi S, Lamont JT. Asymptomatic colonization by *Clostridium difficile* in infants: implications for disease in later life. J Pediatr Gastroenterol Nutr 2010;51:2–7.

73. Eglow R, Pothoulakis C, Itzkowitz S, et al. Diminished *Clostridium difficile* toxin A sensitivity in newborn rabbit ileum is associated with decreased toxin A receptor. J Clin Invest 1992;90:822–9.

74. Stevens V, Dumyati G, Fine LS, et al. Cumulative antibiotic exposures over time and the risk of *Clostridium difficile* infection. Clin Infect Dis 2011;53:42–8.

75. Hensgens MP, Goorhuis A, Dekkers OM, et al. Time interval of increased risk for *Clostridium difficile* infection after exposure to antibiotics. J Antimicrob Chemother 2012;67:742–8.

76. Deshpande A, Pasupuleti V, Thota P, et al. Community-associated *Clostridium difficile* infection and antibiotics: a meta-analysis. J Antimicrob Chemother 2013;68:1951–61.

77. Loo VG, Bourgault AM, Poirier L, et al. Host and pathogen factors for *Clostridium difficile* infection and colonization. N Engl J Med 2011;365:1693–703.

78. Freedberg DE, Salmasian H, Friedman C, et al. Proton pump inhibitors and risk for recurrent *Clostridium difficile* infection among inpatients. Am J Gastroenterol 2013;108:1794–801.

79. Janarthanan S, Ditah I, Adler DG, et al. *Clostridium difficile*-associated diarrhea and proton pump inhibitor therapy: a meta-analysis. Am J Gastroenterol 2012; 107:1001–10.

80. Rogers MA, Greene MT, Young VB, et al. Depression, antidepressant medications, and risk of *Clostridium difficile* infection. BMC Med 2013;11:121.

81. Leung J, Burke B, Ford D, et al. Possible association between obesity and *Clostridium difficile* infection. Emerg Infect Dis 2013;19:1791–8.

82. Bishara J, Farah R, Mograbi J, et al. Obesity as a risk factor for *Clostridium difficile* infection. Clin Infect Dis 2013;57:489–93.

83. Hu MY, Katchar K, Kyne L, et al. Prospective derivation and validation of a clinical prediction rule for recurrent *Clostridium difficile* infection. Gastroenterol 2009;136: 1206–14.

84. Drekonja DM, Amundson WH, Decarolis DD, et al. Antimicrobial use and risk for recurrent *Clostridium difficile* infection. Am J Med 2011;124:1081.e1–7.

85. Bauer MP, Hensgens MP, Miller MA, et al. Renal failure and leukocytosis are predictors of a complicated course of *Clostridium difficile* infection if measured on day of diagnosis. Clin Infect Dis 2012;55(Suppl 2):S149–53.

86. Walk ST, Micic D, Jain R, et al. *Clostridium difficile* ribotype does not predict severe infection. Clin Infect Dis 2012;55:1661–8.

87. Vardakas KZ, Konstantelias AA, Loizidis G, et al. Risk factors for development of *Clostridium difficile* infection due to BI/NAP1/027 strain: a meta-analysis. Int J Infect Dis 2012;16:e768–73.

The Contribution of Strains and Hosts to Outcomes in *Clostridium difficile* Infection

Jessica Martin, MBChB, MRCP

KEYWORDS

- *Clostridium difficile* • Ribotype • Strain • Biomarkers • Risk factors • Mortality
- Recurrence

KEY POINTS

- Molecular typing can be used to identify *Clostridium difficile* strains that are associated with poor clinical outcomes.
- *C difficile* strains that produce binary toxin, in addition to toxins A and B, are associated with an increased risk of recurrence and 30-day mortality.
- Adverse *C difficile* outcomes are associated with increasing age in adults. Children rarely experience severe disease or death caused by *C difficile* infection (CDI).
- High white cell count (WCC), high C-reactive protein (CRP) level, and low serum albumin level are good indicators of CDI severity and are associated with mortality in adults.
- The interactions between strain and host immune response are likely to determine disease susceptibility, severity, and mortality.

INTRODUCTION

Acquisition of *Clostridium difficile* spores can be followed by a spectrum of clinical outcomes ranging from asymptomatic transit through the bowel to severe colitis and death.[1] This clinical variability is a product of bacterial virulence, potentially related to strain type, and host susceptibility to the pathogen. Following germination in the host intestine, *C difficile* can produce 2 cytotoxins: toxin A and toxin B. Some strains produce a third toxin, binary toxin (*C difficile* toxin). The production of these toxins, along with nontoxin virulence factors, and the host's response to them is likely to determine disease severity and clinical outcome. However, measuring strain-related outcomes following *C difficile* infection (CDI) can be challenging because of the high number of strains in most *C difficile* populations and the numerous typing methods used to define them.

University of Leeds, Old Medical School, Leeds General Infirmary, Leeds LS1 3EX, UK
E-mail address: Jessicamartin@nhs.net

Infect Dis Clin N Am 29 (2015) 51–61
http://dx.doi.org/10.1016/j.idc.2014.11.012
0891-5520/15/$ – see front matter © 2015 Elsevier Inc. All rights reserved.

id.theclinics.com

CDI is known to affect vulnerable patients, such as the elderly or immune compromised,[1] but investigating individual host factors can be difficult because of the many variables that influence patients' clinical progress. Large observational studies, using statistical models to adjust for confounders, are required to support links between individual characteristics and outcome measures in order to identify 'high risk' cases of CDI.

The most widely reported CDI outcome measures are recurrence rate and mortality; other measures are reported only sporadically (**Table 1**). Recurrent CDI affects roughly a fifth of patients[2] and is both unpleasant for the individual and a burden on health care resources. Treatments that have recently been introduced, such as fidaxomicin and fecal microbiota transplantation, have been shown to reduce the risk of recurrent CDI.[3,4] Therefore, identification of patients at high risk can help to target these therapies successfully. CDI has been shown to increase mortality, perhaps by 2.5-fold in the 30 days following infection.[5] Even after adjusting for age, sex, and comorbidities, mortality is higher in patients with CDI compared with controls both with and without diarrhea (14.8%, 8.6%, and 5.4%, respectively).[5] This article summarizes recent research into how strain and host factors may be used to identify patients most at risk of disease recurrence and death.

THE INFLUENCE OF STRAIN CHARACTERISTICS ON *CLOSTRIDIUM DIFFICILE* INFECTION OUTCOME
Using Molecular Typing to Predict Clinical Outcomes

Among the many challenges in identifying links between *C difficile* strain type and outcome are the variety of typing methods available, their differing capacities to distinguish between strains, and difficulties in comparing results. Commonly used techniques include (in ascending order of discriminatory power) pulsed-field gel electrophoresis (PFGE), multilocus sequence typing (MLST), polymerase chain reaction ribotyping, restriction endonuclease analysis (REA), and multilocus variable-number tandem-repeat analysis. The emergence of a dominant strain (North American pulsed-field type 1 [NAP1], REA type BI, and ribotype 027, henceforth described as 'ribotype 027') more than a decade ago focused attention on strain-related disease

---

Table 1
Defining outcomes in CDI

Reported CDI Outcomes	
Severe CDI	WCC>15 cells/μL or a serum creatinine level >1.5 times the premorbid level[1]
Complicated CDI	Hypotension, ileus, or megacolon. Some studies include colectomy as complicated CDI[1]
Treatment failure	Heterogeneous definitions are used but this is often defined as failure to achieve symptom resolution after 10 d of treatment. This is difficult to measure retrospectively [end of cell contents][2]
Recurrence	CDI occurring after the completion of treatment for the first episode, often >28 d after diagnosis. Follow-up is usually 60–90 d[2]
ICU admission	—
Interventional surgery	This may be an unreliable outcome measure as surgery may relate to underlying bowel disease or previous surgery, not just CDI
Mortality	Usually 30-d mortality but 14-d to 90-d mortality also reported[2,9]

Abbreviations: ICU, intensive care unit; WCC, white cell count.

severity and mortality, both of which were reportedly increased in patients infected with this strain.[6] More recently, whole-genome sequence analysis has allowed detailed investigation of strains with common ancestors, or shared genes, helping to identify genetic characteristics relevant to clinical outcomes.[7]

Most CDI populations comprise a small number of dominant strains that account for most cases, with the remainder caused by a heterogeneous group of isolates. This diversity, coupled with dominance of the ribotype 027 strain in some Western countries, has led to many studies comparing ribotype 027 with non-027 strains. This approach can be an oversimplification because some of the non-027 strains share key pathologic features with ribotype 027. With this caveat, strain type has been shown to be an important determinant of outcome in most investigations. Following spore acquisition, ribotype 027 is more likely to result in clinical infection than other ribotypes,[8] and multiple studies have linked ribotype 027 with increased severity of infection, recurrence, and mortality.[2,5,6,9–11] The 30-day mortality has been reported as more than twice that of other ribotypes for patients aged 60 to 90 years.[6]

The increase in adverse outcomes associated with ribotype 027 may be caused by several biological features related to its epidemiologic success. The upsurge in this strain occurred in the early 2000s and followed its acquisition of resistance to fluoroquinolone antibiotics.[7] There was high-level use of these antibiotics at the time, especially in areas where ribotype 027 outbreaks were detected, such as North America.[12] Second, this strain produces binary toxin as well as toxins A and B, the presence of which has been associated with poor outcome (**Table 2**).[13] In addition, ribotype 027 has a deletion in the tcdC gene, which has been controversially linked with toxin production.[14] None of these features are unique to ribotype 027, but in combination they are likely to be key to its success.

Using MLST to differentiate *C difficile* populations allows strains to be grouped by common genetic lineage (in clades), unlike when ribotyping is used. However, MLST can still group diverse strains together; for example, clade 1 contains a large

Table 2
Examples of binary toxin *C difficile* strains

Ribotype	Sequence Type (Clade)	Toxins	Comment
027	ST1	A+B+ Binary	Also known as BI or NAP1. Many strains carry the mutation in tcdC.[14] This strain has been associated with increased infection/colonization ratios, and increased recurrence and mortality[2,5,6,9–11]
078	ST11	A+B+ Binary	Common in livestock.[15] Human prevalence of this ribotype is increasing in Europe.[16] This strain has been associated with increased mortality in some studies[2]
023	ST5, ST22	A+B+ Binary	This strain has been associated with increased WCC but not increased mortality.[9] Most contain the tcdC mutation
244	ST41	A+B+ Binary	This strain has been associated with CDI outbreaks in Australia. High associated mortality. TcdC deletion present[21]
066	ST11	A+B+ Binary	This strain has been associated with a similar mortality to ribotypes 027/078[13]
036	ST1	A−B+ Binary	Large deletion in PaLoc leading to reduced transcription of TcdA[22]
033	ST11	A−B− Binary	Rare strains, not associated with symptomatic infection in humans[22]

number of different sequence types.[9] A UK-based study by Walker and colleagues[9] used MLST to investigate 2222 adults with CDI defined according to the detection of toxin. The study showed that sequence type (ST) clade 5 (which contains ribotype 078 strains) was associated with a 14-day mortality of 25%, surpassing that seen (20%) in patients with ST clade 2 (which contains ribotype 027). This observation is important, noting that ribotype 078 strains share many features with ribotype 027, and their prevalence is increasing.[15,16] A Dutch study with a greater representation of ribotype 078 CDI cases did not support the finding of increased mortality compared with other strains (but did show a ribotype 027–related increased mortality).[5] Some studies have not found a link between ribotype 027 and mortality, but lack of power to detect a true association between strain type and outcome is a frequent limitation.[17]

In summary, molecular typing can be used to predict an increased risk of death for patients carrying a small number of common strain types. However, most patients with these strains recover uneventfully and identifying patients at high risk by strain type alone is unlikely to be useful, particularly given that this information is rarely available in a clinically relevant time frame. In the future, identifying specific genetic attributes associated with poor outcome may provide a more specific indicator of which patients are at highest risk. The challenge will be to identify these with sufficient speed to allow timely communication to clinical teams, and then to instigate interventions that can improve outcomes.

Clostridium difficile Toxins and Clostridium difficile Infection Outcomes

Toxigenic *C difficile* strains produce toxins A and B, encoded by tcdA and tcdB in the pathogenicity locus (PaLoc) of the *C difficile* genome.[14] To date, strains lacking these toxins have not been associated with clinical infection and are termed nontoxigenic. The relative significance of toxins A and B to disease severity has been a controversial topic. In the past, toxin A was thought to be the dominant virulence factor in CDI but recent studies using *C difficile* mutants (producing only toxin A or B) have shown that toxin B, but not toxin A, is essential for disease.[18] This is supported by reports of clinical outbreaks caused by A−/B+ strains (eg, ribotype 017),[10] which have been associated with similar outcomes to strains producing both toxins.[2] Toxins A and B have direct cytotoxic effects on intestinal epithelial cells and provoke inflammatory responses leading to tissue damage.[14] High cytotoxin titers in feces have been shown to correlate positively with increased symptom severity.[19]

In addition to toxins A and B, a small number of strains produce binary toxin, encoded at a site distant to the PaLoc (see **Table 2**).[20] Binary toxin is associated with increased CDI mortality, regardless of ribotype,[13,14] and has been shown in some studies to be an independent risk factor for CDI recurrence.[20] A recently described Australian outbreak was caused by a binary toxin–producing strain, ribotype 244.[21] This strain was associated with higher mortality than others, with a high odds ratio of 13.5. However, the presence of binary toxin genes does not necessarily mean that the toxin is produced in vivo; there are currently no binary toxin detection assays in routine laboratory use.[22] A large UK study found that binary toxin–producing strains in clade 3 (ribotype 023) were associated with increased white cell count (WCC) and C-reactive protein but not mortality.[9] It can be deduced that binary toxin has a role in pathogenesis but the presence of binary toxin genes alone cannot be correlated directly with CDI outcome. Further studies measuring binary toxin levels in stool may be informative.

A missense mutation in tcdC is present in some *C difficile* strains.[14] It has been shown to play a role in toxin A/B regulation[14] and it was thought to explain high virulence by increasing toxin production in some strains, such as ribotype 027. However, the presence of this mutation is not universally associated with severe disease; *tcdC* functional state does not relate to severity when covariates are adjusted for.[23,24] Strains shown to produce excess toxin similarly do not always have a mutation in *tcdC*, and therefore other factors must be important in the regulation of toxin production.[14]

Several investigations have attempted to tease out the relative importance of *C difficile* virulence factors. A UK study differentiated patients by tcdC mutation and binary toxin genes.[25] tcdC-containing strains were associated with increased CRP and WCC but not poor outcome, whereas binary toxin producers were associated with high WCC and higher 30-day mortality (31% vs 14% in binary toxin–negative strains). However, the number of tcdC-containing isolates in this study was small. Other studies have investigated strain type, tcdC deletion, and binary toxin status and did not find an association with mortality, concluding that host factors may be more important than strain.[22,26] It is clear that further studies investigating toxin titers in vivo, and toxin regulation, would help to improve understanding of how *C difficile* toxins relate to recurrence and CDI mortality.

Nontoxin Virulence Factors

To cause clinical disease, *C difficile* spores must interact with host epithelial tissue, germinate, and produce toxins (**Fig. 1**). Sporulation is also required for onward transmission via the fecal-oral route. Many known and unknown virulence factors facilitate these biochemical processes but little is known about the differential ability of *C difficile* strains to produce them.

The surface layer (S layer) is the outermost protein layer of *C difficile*, is responsible for adhesion to host tissue, and is known to be variable between strains.[14] A study investigating animal and human isolates showed that variation in the S layer led to variable adherence to epithelial cells.[27] Thus, the success of intestinal colonization and infection is likely to relate to surface proteins. It is known that immune evasion by *C difficile* is also important.[14]

Given that clostridial spores are the main mode of transmission, it seems logical that virulent strains produce spores in greater numbers, or possibly more resilient spores. This theory has not been consistently shown in vitro; for example, in one study, ribotype 027 strains had a lower sporulation rate than other strains.[25] SpoOA has been identified as the master regulator of sporulation, and has been implicated in toxin gene expression and biofilm formation (in mice).[28] It may also be relevant to the regulation of other virulence factors (eg, flagella).[14] Experiments suggest that SpoOA-associated regulation of toxin production may vary between ribotypes but further work is required before clinical conclusions can be drawn.[29]

THE INFLUENCE OF HOST CHARACTERISTICS ON *CLOSTRIDIUM DIFFICILE* INFECTION OUTCOME

CDI typically affects older patients, often with recent hospital contact, who have received antibiotic treatment. Recent changes in CDI epidemiology, with a greater number of patients presenting in community settings, have shown an increase in CDI in younger patients, some of whom have not been exposed to antibiotics.[30] New technologies, such as whole-genome sequencing, allow detailed analysis of intestinal flora and have led to a greater understanding of the changes in host microbiota relating to CDI susceptibility,[31] perhaps explaining some of these epidemiologic changes. Many host factors have been linked to CDI risk and adverse outcomes, and the current evidence is summarized later.

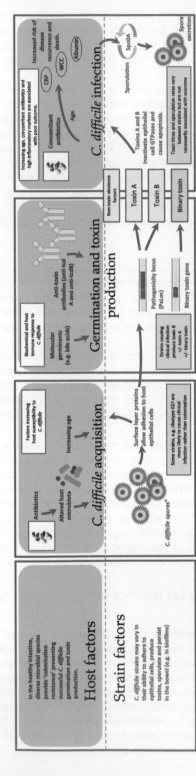

Fig. 1. Host and strain influences on *C difficile* germination, toxin production, and sporulation. CRP, C-reactive protein; WCC, peripheral white cell count. [a] Not accurate in morphology or scale.

Age

The risk of a poor outcome from CDI is closely related to patient age. Older patients (>65 years) are more likely to have recurrent CDI and have a greater risk of death in the weeks following infection compared with younger individuals.[2,6,32,33] CDI-related mortality increases at a rate of roughly 2% per year of adult life.[2,32,33] It was suggested that a weak immune response to C difficile toxin in elderly patients is the reason for poor outcome, although a recent study showed that antitoxin antibody responses were independent of age.[26]

In children, C difficile colonization is common, especially in the first year of life,[34] but severe infection and death are much less common than in the adult population.[35] The reasons for this are not entirely understood. In contrast with adult patients, in whom renal function and WCC are linked to clinical outcome, there are no clear predictors of disease severity or death in children[35]; adequately sized and controlled studies in children are needed. Understanding the main differences in the biochemical and immune responses to C difficile between young and old may provide valuable clues about why age remains an independent risk factor for poor CDI outcome.

Antibiotics and Intestinal Microbiota

In health, gut microbes provide protection from pathogens; this is known as colonization resistance. In response to C difficile, the normal human microbiome is thought to inactivate germinant molecules, thus preventing intraluminal germination and disease.[14] The intestinal environment has also been shown to prevent inappropriate inflammation of gut epithelium in response to low-level C difficile, suggesting a link between host microbiota and regulation of disease severity once germination has occurred.[14,36] Hospital patients have been shown to have fewer bacterial groups in their intestinal flora than healthy volunteers,[36] regardless of C difficile status, perhaps going some way to explaining the origins of CDI as a health care–associated infection. A small study showed no difference between the fecal microbiota of asymptomatic C difficile carriers and healthy subjects, but lower bacterial diversity in patients with C difficile–related diarrhea.[37]

Antibiotics predispose patients to CDI by disruption of the host microflora allowing germination and proliferation of C difficile. CDI risk increases 6-fold during antibiotic treatment and for the month that follows.[2,38] All antibiotics are associated with CDI but cephalosporins, fluoroquinolones, and clindamycin carry the greatest risk, although interactions between strain type and antibiotic choice may be important. As mentioned earlier, fluoroquinolone use has been associated with an increased risk of ribotype 027.[10] Susceptibility to ribotype 017 infection has been linked to clindamycin treatment, but this strain is not commonly resistant to clindamycin[10] and so its CDI disposition presumably relates more to antibiotic-mediated effects on the microbiome.

The use of antibiotics for other infections following the onset of CDI (concomitant antibiotics) increases the risk of recurrent infection and disease-related death,[2,32,33] especially if antibiotics are started after CDI treatment has finished.[33] The recovery of the microbial environment following CDI is important in reducing the risk of recurrent infection, and ongoing antibiotic treatment perpetuates host bacterial imbalance.[35] A decrease in the phylum Bacteroidetes has been associated with recurrent CDI[39] but it is likely that the combination of microbial groups, rather than the presence of absence of one species, is important in the acquisition and recurrence of CDI.[40] Replenishment of normal bacterial diversity, using fecal microbiota transplantation, has been successful in patients with multiple recurrences.[3]

Immune Response

The presence of C difficile toxins in the intestinal lumen stimulates a multifaceted immune response involving cytokines, chemokines, and mucosal immune cells.[14] Antitoxin antibodies (anti-TcdA and anti-TcdB) are important in determining whether colonization or clinical infection follows C difficile spore acquisition.[26] Reduced anti-TcdA levels at the start of infection have been linked to both recurrence and an increased 30-day mortality.[2,26] Investigation into the role of antibodies to toxin B has been less conclusive,[26] so the precise relationship between antitoxin antibodies and disease severity is yet to be fully elucidated.

Surface layer proteins (SLPs) are present in all C difficile isolates, and anti-SLP antibodies are readily recovered from the serum of patients with CDI. SLPs induce cytokine production and stimulate monocyte-derived dendritic cells.[14,27] The host gut also produces anti-microbial peptides to protect itself against C difficile, genes conferring resistance to these peptides have been isolated from some C difficile strains. Thus, the interaction between pathogen and host immune response is closely linked to disease severity and mortality[14] in patients with CDI and research is now being performed on immunotherapies, such as monoclonal antibodies to C difficile toxins, for the treatment of CDI.

Biomarkers

Biological markers, especially WCC but also CRP, serum creatinine, and albumin concentrations, have been reported to be associated with CDI severity and are possible independent predictors of mortality.[2,9,17,26,32] These markers accounted for 30% to 40% of the MLST clade–related mortality in one UK study,[9] suggesting that inflammatory processes have a greater influence on poor outcome than strain type alone. However, these biomarkers are nonspecific to C difficile disease. Fecal lactoferrin and interleukin-8 are produced in response to C difficile toxins and have been investigated as predictors of CDI disease severity.[41,42] They can readily be measured in stool samples and one study showed that patients with clinically severe CDI have fecal lactoferrin levels 5-fold greater than in mild/moderation infection.[42] Further clinical studies are required to define CDI-specific biomarkers for prospective clinical use.

Other Clinical Variables

Measures of comorbidities, such as the Charlson comorbidity index, are included in many studies on CDI outcome but mixed conclusions have been drawn.[10,17,20,32,33] A recent systematic review concluded that comorbidities increase the risk of mortality from CDI.[2]

The relationship between proton pump inhibitor (PPI) use and CDI has been debated for many years. There are several studies linking PPI use to recurrence[2] but there are few data on the indications for acid suppression in patients with CDI, or the risk of adverse events (eg, intestinal bleeding) resulting from PPI cessation. From a clinical point of view, PPIs would ideally be stopped in patients with CDI but a case-by-case risk assessment is required based on the indication for use.

SUMMARY

CDI continues to be associated with significant morbidity rates and mortality rates. Using strain and host factors to identify high-risk patients helps to target health care resources effectively. However, only a small number of strains have been associated with adverse outcome and using strain type to predict CDI outcome lacks specificity. In the future, genomic analysis may be able to identify specific genetic attributes relating to poor outcome. The challenge is in being able to identify high-risk individuals in a clinically relevant time frame.

Biomarkers such as WCC, CRP, and albumin are closely associated with CDI mortality and are easy to measure in routine clinical practice. Recent data support their use in the risk assessment of patients with CDI but increasing age and comorbidities remain as poor prognostic indicators. Overall, it can be concluded that a single strain or host variable cannot be used to determine the clinical outcome of CDI. Instead, a complex pathologic pathway determined by toxigenic and nontoxigenic virulence factors, and moderated by the host intestinal environment and immune response, determines the clinical outcome for each patient with CDI.

REFERENCES

1. Cohen SH, Dolin R, Blaser MJ, et al. Clinical practice guidelines for *Clostridium difficile* infection in adults: 2010 update by the Society for Healthcare Epidemiology of America (SHEA) and the Infectious Diseases Society of America (IDSA). Infect Control Hosp Epidemiol 2010;31(5):431–55.
2. Abou Chakra CN, Pepin J, Sirard S, et al. Risk factors for recurrence, complications and mortality in *Clostridium difficile* infection: a systematic review. PLoS One 2014;9(6):e98400.
3. van Nood E, Vrieze A, Nieuwdorp M, et al. Duodenal infusion of donor feces for recurrent *Clostridium difficile*. N Engl J Med 2013;368(5):407–15.
4. Cornely OA, Crook DW, Esposito R, et al. Fidaxomicin versus vancomycin for infection with *Clostridium difficile* in Europe, Canada, and the USA: a double-blind, non-inferiority, randomised controlled trial. Lancet Infect Dis 2012;12(4):281–9.
5. Hensgens MP, Goorhuis A, Dekker OM, et al. All-cause and disease-specific mortality in hospitalized patients with *Clostridium difficile* infection: a multicenter cohort study. Clin Infect Dis 2013;56(8):1108–16.
6. Miller M, Gravel D, Mulvey M, et al. Health care-associated *Clostridium difficile* infection in Canada: patient age and infecting strain type are highly predictive of severe outcome and mortality. Clin Infect Dis 2010;50(2):194–201.
7. He M, Miyajima F, Roberts P, et al. Emergence and global spread of epidemic healthcare-associated *Clostridium difficile*. Nat Genet 2013;45:109–13.
8. Loo VG, Bourgault AM, Poirier L, et al. Host and pathogen factors for *Clostridium difficile* infection and colonization. N Engl J Med 2011;365(18):1693–703.
9. Walker AS, Eyre DW, Wyllie D, et al. Relationship between bacterial strain type, host biomarkers, and mortality in *Clostridium difficile* infection. Clin Infect Dis 2013;56(11):1589–600.
10. Goorhuis A, Debast SB, Dutilh JC, et al. Type-specific risk factors and outcome in an outbreak with 2 different *Clostridium difficile* types simultaneously in 1 hospital. Clin Infect Dis 2011. http://dx.doi.org/10.1093/cid/cir549.
11. See I, Mu Y, Cohen J, et al. NAP1 strain type predicts outcomes from *Clostridium difficile* infection. Clin Infect Dis 2014;58(10):1394–400.
12. Warny M, Pepin J, Fang A, et al. Toxin production by an emerging strain of *Clostridium difficile* associated with outbreaks of severe disease in North America and Europe. Lancet 2005;366(9491):1079–84.
13. Bacci S, Molbak K, Kjeldsen MK, et al. Binary toxin and death after *Clostridium difficile* infection. Emerg Infect Dis 2011;17(6):976.
14. Vedantam G, Clark A, Chu M, et al. *Clostridium difficile* infection: toxins and nontoxin virulence factors, and their contributions to disease establishment and host response. Gut Microbes 2012;3(2):121–34.

15. Goorhuis A, Bakker D, Corver J, et al. Emergence of *Clostridium difficile* infection due to a new hypervirulent strain, polymerase chain reaction ribotype 078. Clin Infect Dis 2008;47(9):1162–70.
16. Public Health England. *Clostridium difficile* ribotyping network for England and Northern Ireland 2011-2013 report. Available at: https://www.gov.uk/government/uploads/system/uploads/attachment_data/file/329156/C_difficile_ribotyping_network_CDRN_report.pdf. Accessed August 31, 2014.
17. Walk ST, Micic D, Jain R, et al. *Clostridium difficile* ribotype does not predict severe infection. Clin Infect Dis 2012. http://dx.doi.org/10.1093/cid/cis786.
18. Carter GP, Julian IR, Lyras D. The role of toxin A and toxin B in the virulence of *Clostridium difficile*. Trends Microbiol 2012;20(1):21–9.
19. Åkerlund T, Svenungsson B, Lagergren A, et al. Correlation of disease severity with fecal toxin levels in patients with *Clostridium difficile*-associated diarrhea and distribution of PCR ribotypes and toxin yields in vitro of corresponding isolates. J Clin Microbiol 2006;44(2):353–8.
20. Stewart DB, Berg A, Hegarty J. Predicting recurrence of *C. difficile* colitis using bacterial virulence factors: binary toxin is the key. J Gastrointest Surg 2013; 17(1):118–25.
21. Lim SK, Stuart RL, Mackin K, et al. Emergence of a ribotype 244 strain of *Clostridium difficile* associated with severe disease and related to the epidemic ribotype 027 strain. Clin Infect Dis 2014. http://dx.doi.org/10.1093/cid/ciu203.
22. Gerding DN, Johnson S, Rupnik M, et al. *Clostridium difficile* binary toxin CDT: mechanism, epidemiology, and potential clinical importance. Gut Microbes 2013;5(1):6–18.
23. Cartman ST, Kelly ML, Heeg D, et al. Precise manipulation of the *Clostridium difficile* chromosome reveals a lack of association between the tcdC genotype and toxin production. Appl Environ Microbiol 2012;78(13):4683–90.
24. Goldenberg SD, French GL. Lack of association of *tcdC* type and binary toxin status with disease severity and outcome in toxigenic *Clostridium difficile*. J Infect 2011;62(5):355–62.
25. Sirard S, Valiquette L, Fortier L. Lack of association between clinical outcome of *Clostridium difficile* infections, strain type, and virulence-associated phenotypes. J Clin Microbiol 2011;49(12):4040–6.
26. Solomon K, Martin AJ, O'Donoghue C, et al. Mortality in patients with *Clostridium difficile* infection correlates with host pro-inflammatory and humoral immune responses. J Med Microbiol 2013;62(Pt 9):1453–60.
27. Spigaglia P, Barketi-Klai A, Collignon A, et al. Surface-layer (S-layer) of human and animal *Clostridium difficile* strains and their behaviour in adherence to epithelial cells and intestinal colonization. J Med Microbiol 2013;62(Pt 9):1386–93.
28. Pettit LJ, Browne HP, Yu L, et al. Functional genomics reveals that *Clostridium difficile* Spo0A coordinates sporulation, virulence and metabolism. BMC Genomics 2014;15(1):160.
29. Mackin KE, Carter GP, Howarth P, et al. Spo0A differentially regulates toxin production in evolutionarily diverse strains of *Clostridium difficile*. PLoS One 2013; 8(11):e79666.
30. Wilcox MH, Mooney L, Bendall R, et al. A case-control study of community-associated *Clostridium difficile* infection. J Antimicrob Chemother 2008;62(2): 388–96.
31. Shankar V, Hamilton MJ, Khoruts A, et al. Species and genus level resolution analysis of gut microbiota in *Clostridium difficile* patients following fecal microbiota transplantation. Microbiome 2014;2(1):13.

32. Rodríguez-Pardo D, Almirante B, Bartolome R, et al. Epidemiology of *Clostridium difficile* infection and risk factors for unfavorable clinical outcomes: results of a hospital-based study in Barcelona, Spain. J Clin Microbiol 2013;51(5):1465–73.
33. Zilberberg MD, Reske K, Olsen M, et al. Risk factors for recurrent *Clostridium difficile* infection (CDI) hospitalization among hospitalized patients with an initial CDI episode: a retrospective cohort study. BMC Infect Dis 2014;14:306.
34. Rousseau C, Poilane I, De Pontual L, et al. *Clostridium difficile* carriage in healthy infants in the community: a potential reservoir for pathogenic strains. Clin Infect Dis 2012;55:1209–15.
35. Schwartz KL, Darwish I, Richardson SE, et al. Severe clinical outcome is uncommon in *Clostridium difficile* infection in children: a retrospective cohort study. BMC Pediatr 2014;14(1):28.
36. Skraban J, Dzeroski S, Zenko B, et al. Gut microbiota patterns associated with colonization of different *Clostridium difficile* ribotypes. PLoS One 2013;8(2): e58005.
37. Rea MC, O'Sullivan O, Shanahan F, et al. *Clostridium difficile* carriage in elderly subjects and associated changes in the intestinal microbiota. J Clin Microbiol 2012;50(3):867–75.
38. Hensgens MP, Goorhuis A, Dekkers OM, et al. Time interval of increased risk for *Clostridium difficile* infection after exposure to antibiotics. J Antimicrob Chemother 2012;67(3):742–8.
39. Chang JY, Antonopoulos DA, Kalra A, et al. Decreased diversity of the fecal microbiome in recurrent *Clostridium difficile*-associated diarrhea. J Infect Dis 2008; 197(3):435–8.
40. Lawley TD, Claire S, Walker AW, et al. Targeted restoration of the intestinal microbiota with a simple, defined bacteriotherapy resolves relapsing *Clostridium difficile* disease in mice. PLoS Pathog 2012;8(10):e1002995.
41. Boone JH, Archbald-Pannone LR, Wickham KN, et al. Ribotype 027 *Clostridium difficile* infections with measurable stool toxin have increased lactoferrin and are associated with a higher mortality. Eur J Clin Microbiol Infect Dis 2014;33(6): 1045–51.
42. Boone JH, DiPersio JR, Tan MJ, et al. Elevated lactoferrin is associated with moderate to severe *Clostridium difficile* disease, stool toxin, and 027 infection. Eur J Clin Microbiol Infect Dis 2013;32(12):1517–23.

Diagnostic Pitfalls in *Clostridium difficile* Infection

Tim Planche, MD, FRCPath[a], Mark H. Wilcox, MD, FRCPath[b],*

KEYWORDS

- *Clostridium difficile* • Diagnostic accuracy • Cytotoxin assay
- Nucleic acid amplification test • Immunoassay • Culture

KEY POINTS

- Clinical differentiation of *Clostridium difficile* infection (CDI) from other causes of hospital-acquired diarrhea is poor, making laboratory diagnosis an important intervention.
- Diagnostic strategies that only test on physician request underestimate the prevalence of *C difficile*.
- Laboratory tests for *C difficile* broadly detect either the organism or its toxins. Tests that detect organism are more frequently positive than those targeting toxin. However, detection of free toxin in feces better identifies patients with clinical disease and so has advantages for disease diagnosis.
- Rapid tests such as nucleic acid amplification tests or immunoassays are available for results within hours, compared with several days for conventional reference assays.
- Two-stage or 3-stage testing algorithms improve the diagnostic accuracy for CDI.

INTRODUCTION: NATURE OF THE PROBLEM

Clostridium difficile is an anaerobic, spore-forming, Gram-positive bacillus, and is a leading cause of infectious diarrhea, particularly in hospitalized patients receiving antimicrobial therapy.[1,2] After overgrowth in the colon, *C difficile* produces 2 enterotoxins, *C difficile* toxin (CDT) A and CDT B, which cause diarrhea. CDT is encoded by the tcdA and tcdB genes on the PaLoc region.[3] Not all strains of *C difficile* possess the PaLoc region and produce CDT, and these nontoxigenic strains of *C difficile* do not cause disease.[4] It is important to differentiate nontoxigenic strains from the potentially pathogenic toxigenic bacteria; however, the presence of the toxigenic strains is not synonymous with CDI, as these bacteria may harmlessly colonize individuals. Furthermore,

---

[a] Division of Cellular and Molecular Medicine, Centre for Infection, University of London, St. George's Hospital, Cranmer Terrace, London SW17 0RE, UK; [b] Microbiology, University of Leeds, Leeds Teaching Hospitals, Old Medical School, Leeds General Infirmary, West Yorkshire, Leeds LS1 3EX, UK
* Corresponding author.
E-mail address: Mark.Wilcox@leedsth.nhs.uk

Infect Dis Clin N Am 29 (2015) 63–82
http://dx.doi.org/10.1016/j.idc.2014.11.008
0891-5520/15/$ – see front matter © 2015 Elsevier Inc. All rights reserved.

id.theclinics.com

patients colonized with *C difficile* may be significantly less likely to develop CDI than noncolonized individuals, probably because of the development of protective antibodies in the former.[5,6]

Approximately 3000 and 14-20,000 deaths attributable to CDI are reported annually in the United Kingdom and United States, respectively.[2,7] There is an attributable case fatality rate of 6% to 17%,[8–12] with the elderly at greatest risk.[8,10,13,14] Accurate diagnosis is essential for the management of individual patients and the control of infection, but also so that the true efficacy of interventions can be evaluated and to provide reliable epidemiologic data. This article discusses not only the available methods for the diagnosis of CDI but also who and when to test, and the interpretation of results.

Hospital associated diarrhea is a very common symptom with many underlying causes, both infectious and noninfectious, which are outlined in **Box 1**; for example, in a United States university teaching hospital, 60 of 485 (12%) hospitalized patients reported 2 or more loose, unformed stools in the last 24 hours.[15] Depending on the setting and case definition, CDI is responsible for 4% to 30% of diarrhea samples sent to the laboratory.[12,16–20] The clinical differentiation of CDI from other causes is not possible with any great reliability, especially as those at greatest risk are also

---

Box 1
Common causes of diarrhea

Infectious Causes

Clostridium difficile

Norovirus

Other viruses: rotavirus, adenovirus

Other bacteria: *Salmonella, Campylobacter, Shigella, Escherichia coli*

Noninfectious Causes

Inflammatory bowel disease

Gastrointestinal neoplasia

Irritable bowel syndrome

Celiac disease

Anxiety

Food allergy

Lactose intolerance

Iatrogenic Causes

Use of laxatives

Nasogastric feeding

Post–gastrointestinal surgery

Radiotherapy

Antibiotic-associated diarrhea (noninfective)

Other drugs, selective serotonin reuptake inhibitors, nonsteroidal anti-inflammatory drugs, statins

more likely to have other causes of diarrhea (medical, surgical, and iatrogenic); thus, accurate laboratory diagnosis of CDI is essential.

The consequences of false-negative laboratory results are well recognized, as they lead to patients not being treated for CDI; in addition, if clinicians lose confidence in test accuracy, increased use of empiric CDI therapy may occur, ironically potentially leading to overtreatment and possibly risk of (true) CDI secondary to further gut microbiome perturbation. Conversely, it is less often appreciated that there are potentially serious consequences of false-positive results. False-positive CDI results may mean that alternative diagnoses are no longer considered, and appropriate antibiotics are stopped or substituted with inappropriate alternatives. Patients labeled incorrectly as having CDI may consume valuable infection isolation resources and capacity, with knock-on effects for other transmissible infections/pathogens. Moreover, the strategy of cohorting together patients with false-positive results onto isolation wards for *C difficile* could expose these patients to an increased risk of acquiring genuine CDI. Again, inappropriate CDI treatment may theoretically exacerbate risk of (true) *C difficile* disease.

PATHOGENESIS

The pathogenesis and course of CDI is summarized in **Fig. 1**. First, the potential host is exposed to *C difficile* spores of a toxigenic strain of *C difficile*. Next there is overgrowth of the *C difficile*, which normally occurs after disruption of normal bowel flora by antibiotic therapy. Alternatively, patients may become temporarily colonized or enter a carrier state. Finally, there needs to be toxin production that results in CDI, usually manifested as diarrhea. Different stages of the development of CDI will have either organism present or detectable free toxin, or both. This process has important potential implications for the diagnostic tests.

EPIDEMIOLOGY

An understanding of the epidemiology of *C difficile*, particularly with regard to the detection of toxin or bacteria, is necessary to understand CDI diagnosis. Toxigenic *C difficile* may be found in the stool of otherwise healthy patients without diarrhea. Toxigenic *C difficile* was cultured from the feces of 2% healthy Swedish or British adults,[21,22] without detectable free CDT in feces. Higher rates of toxigenic *C difficile* are generally found in patients admitted to hospital. Toxigenic *C difficile* may be found in 10% to 24% of asymptomatic hospital admissions,[23,24] and recent hospitalization is a risk factor for the detection of *C difficile* in asymptomatic patients.[25] After admission, toxigenic *C difficile* may be found in the feces of up to 20% to 30% of asymptomatic adults who have been inpatients for several weeks.[23,25,26] As diarrhea is such a common symptom, it is clearly possible that a patient with diarrhea not attributable to CDI can have *C difficile* present as a 'bystander' organism. Thus, reliance on detecting the presence of *C difficile* in patients with such a common symptom may overestimate the true incidence of CDI.

REFERENCE TESTS

As with any disease or condition, the assessment of a new laboratory test to confirm to CDI depends on the reference standard assay (gold standard) with which it is compared. A key difficulty here is that there are 2 reference assays for *C difficile*, each detecting different targets (see later discussion). Use of the wrong reference assay can falsely reassure on diagnostic accuracy. This aspect is particularly important in CDI where detection of *C difficile* in asymptomatic patients is common, and tests detecting the presence of *C difficile* may overcall true CDI.

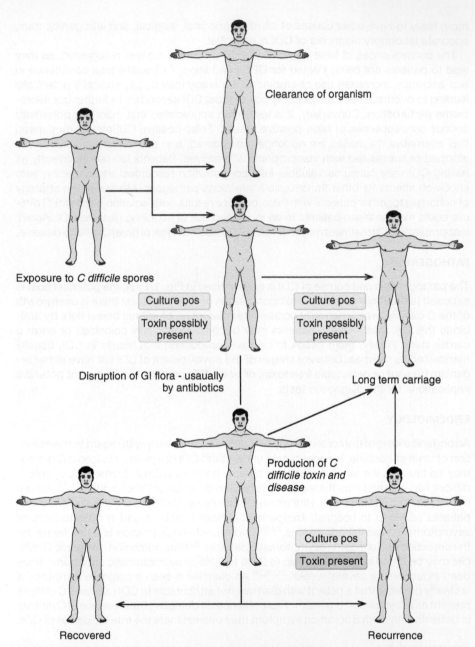

Clearance of organism

Exposure to *C difficile* spores

Culture pos

Toxin possibly present

Culture pos

Toxin possibly present

Disruption of GI flora - usually by antibiotics

Long term carriage

Producion of *C difficile* toxin and disease

Culture pos

Toxin present

Recovered

Recurrence

Fig. 1. Acquisition of *Clostridium difficile*. GI, gastrointestinal.

One *C difficile* reference assay, the cell cytotoxicity assay (CCTA), measures the presence of free toxin in feces, whereas the other, cytotoxigenic culture (CC), detects the presence of the organism, or more precisely, the presence of bacteria (usually spores) that can produce toxins. The methodologies for these tests are shown in **Figs. 2** and **3**. CCTA relies on the detection of the cytopathic effect in cell culture (**Fig. 4**) that is neutralized by the presence of antibodies to CDT (or *Clostridium sordelli*

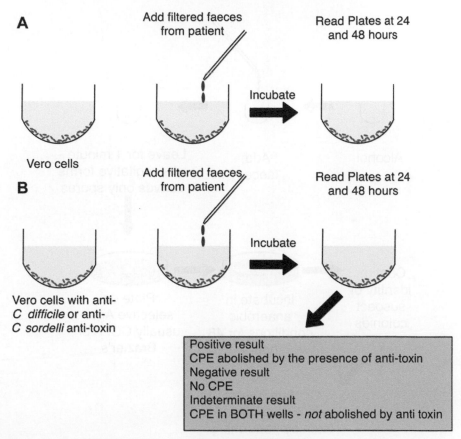

A Add filtered faeces from patient

Read Plates at 24 and 48 hours

Vero cells

Incubate

B Add filtered faeces from patient

Read Plates at 24 and 48 hours

Incubate

Vero cells with anti-*C difficile* or anti-*C sordelli* anti-toxin

Positive result
CPE abolished by the presence of anti-toxin
Negative result
No CPE
Indeterminate result
CPE in BOTH wells - *not* abolished by anti toxin

Fig. 2. (*A, B*) Cell cytotoxicity assay. CPE, cytopathic effect.

toxin). Cells (usually Vero cells) are cultured in the presence of stool filtrate with and without the presence of antitoxin antibodies. These cultures are examined microscopically at 24 and 48 hours for a cytopathic effect that is abolished by antitoxin. This test requires the ability to perform cell culture, which is rarely used now in laboratories (although maintaining a semicontinuous cell line should be within the scope of most microbiology laboratories). There is also variation in the exact methodologies described for CCTA, with variation in the cell lines used, the filtration and dilution of feces, and antibody [27–30] Although most positive results are available by 24 hours, negative results may take a further 24 hours to become available.

CC relies on the culture of *C difficile* from stool (**Fig. 5**), which is usually first exposed to alcohol shock to remove bacteria, other than the alcohol-resistant spores of *C difficile*. As there are nontoxigenic *C difficile* strains, it is necessary to confirm that cultured isolates produce toxin in vitro. As with CCTA, there are also variations in the exact methodologies used for CC, with differences in the culture conditions and the way *C difficile* is identified, how and whether alcohol shock is performed, and how in vitro toxin production is detected.[31–36] CC may take up to 5 days to produce a result.

Several studies have compared the performance of CCTA and CC, and it is clear that CC detects more positive samples than CCTA; CCTA detects about 15% to 40% fewer '*C difficile* cases' than CC.[12,16,18,19,37–41] More rarely, specimens (2%–

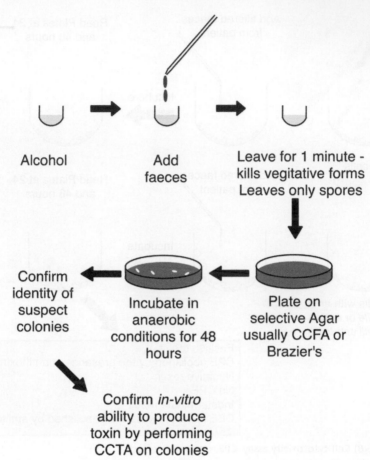

Alcohol

Add faeces

Leave for 1 minute - kills vegitative forms Leaves only spores

Confirm identity of suspect colonies

Incubate in anaerobic conditions for 48 hours

Plate on selective Agar usually CCFA or Brazier's

Confirm *in-vitro* ability to produce toxin by performing CCTA on colonies

Fig. 3. Cytotoxigenic culture. CCFA, cycloserine-cefoxitin-fructose agar; CCTA, cell cytotoxicity assay.

15%) are found that are CC negative but positive by CCTA. The level of agreement of these tests is intermediate, with reported κ values of 0.7 to 0.9. Thus, it is clear that these reference assays are performing differently and are not interchangeable. As CC is more frequently positive, and because CCTA has perceived technical difficulties (the need for cell culture), some consider CC as the 'true' gold-standard test for CDI.[42] However, as these assays have different targets, their lack of agreement is not surprising. Detection of more positive samples may simply mean more false-positives and does not necessarily mean that a test is better per se. Clinical validation of the tests is needed to resolve the controversy.

CLINICAL VALIDATION OF TESTS FOR *CLOSTRIDIUM DIFFICILE* INFECTION

Large studies are required for the robust clinical validation of a test. It is noteworthy, however, that typical studies on diagnostic tests involve small or moderate sample sizes. Underpowered studies can produce misleading estimates and may fail to reveal true differences between the accuracy of diagnostic tests. Crucially, diagnostic evaluations usually do not include clinical outcome data; as such, the assumption is that the test(s) being examined are detecting a clinically relevant disease or target.

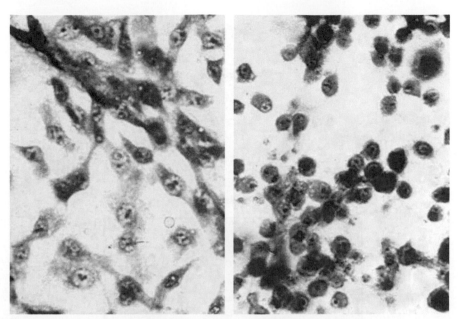

Fig. 4. (*Left*) Cytopathic effect on Vero cells: normal cells. (*Right*) Cells exhibiting cytopathic effects (cell rounding) caused by *C difficile* toxin (staining = methylene blue).

An early study in the 1980s showed that patients with diarrheal samples that yielded positive CCTA results had worse outcomes and indicators of severity compared with controls without diarrhea.[43] By contrast, patients who were *C difficile* culture positive but who had a negative CCTA were indistinguishable from controls in terms of outcomes. Colonoscopy was performed on about 70% of the patients, and showed much higher rates of pseudomembranous colitis (51% vs 11%) in CCTA-positive cases in comparison with those who were culture positive but CCTA negative. Other small studies conducted around the same time comparing the results of endoscopy with those of reference assays showed that nearly all patients with pseudomembranous colitis were CCTA positive.[44,45]

Another small study (from 1986) followed 29 patients with diarrhea who were CC positive but CCTA negative, and not treated for CDI.[46] Most of these patients recovered spontaneously without the need for any treatment of CDI, or had alternative diagnoses proven. These early studies, despite being relatively underpowered, were consistent with the CCTA being a better predictor of disease and, given the longer time to results for CC, meant that CCTA became the preferred CDI diagnostic and reference method. The introduction in the 1990s of enzyme immunoassays for CDTs (toxEIAs) led many laboratories to abandon CCTA in favor of these more rapid and less labor-intensive tests. Subsequent dissatisfaction with the accuracy of toxEIAs (both suboptimal sensitivity and specificity; see later discussion) meant that high-sensitivity test alternatives were sought. In particular, the advent of rapid commercial nucleic acid amplification tests (NAATs) for *C difficile*, which detected increased numbers of positive samples, led to an increased acceptance of CC (which best correlated with NAATs) as a reference standard for CDI.[42]

Recently a multicenter study of CDI, the largest ever to be performed, has clinically validated the results of 12,420 fecal samples.[12] This study examined the results of the 2 reference assays (CC and CCTA) for all diarrheal stool samples sent to 4 diagnostic

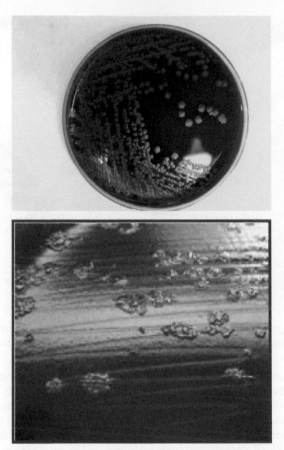

Fig. 5. Appearance of typical colonies of *C difficile*.

laboratories, in addition to those for 4 commercial CDI tests; the results were compared with outcome and clinical and laboratory data. The 6522 inpatients were assessed in 3 groups: CCTA positive (group 1); CC positive and CCTA negative (*C difficile* colonized/excretors, group 2); and negative by all tests (negative controls, group 3). All-cause 30-day mortality was markedly and significantly higher in group 1 than in group 2 (72 of 435 [16.6%] vs 20 of 207 [9.7%] patients; *P* = .022), showing that detection of toxin in feces (CCTA) best correlates with severe clinical outcome. Of note, the rate of all-cause mortality in *C difficile*–negative patients with diarrhea (group 3: 503 of 5880, 8.6%), was not significantly different from the death rate in patients with a positive CC-only result. The high observed mortality rate in patients with diarrhea but no diagnostic evidence of CDI (which indeed is higher than the 30-day[47] or 60-day[48] in-hospital death rates for myocardial infarction) highlights the need for inclusion of *C difficile*–negative controls with diarrhea in clinical validation studies. These findings were confirmed in a multivariate analysis. Furthermore, a similar pattern was seen when comparing other outcome measures such as hospital stay or markers of severity (white blood cell count, albumin, serum creatinine); these were all significantly higher in group 1, but no different between groups 2 and 3. Further clinical information was available in patients with positive CC but negative CCTA; such fatal cases did not have a diagnosis of CDI recorded on their death certificates, only 12% had a clinical diagnosis of CDI recorded in their clinical records, and only 55% had diarrhea recorded. Finally, as this was an observational study, 75 patients who were CC positive but CCTA negative did not receive any specific therapy for CDI; of note, these had a lower mortality rate (4 of 75, 5%) than the *C difficile*–negative controls.

The findings of this large outcomes-based study clearly validate CCTA as the best diagnostic indicator of CDI as a disease. However, a positive CC may still indicate a patient who is an infection risk to others on the ward. In effect, the 2 tests may be answering different questions: CCTA indicates whether diarrheal symptoms are due to CDI, whereas CC-positive but CCTA-negative patients are unlikely to have CDI, although these individuals may represent an infection risk to others as they are excreting toxigenic *C difficile.* Several more recent smaller studies have shown similar results.[49–51] Although these studies used commercial assays (see later discussion), they broadly confirm that toxin detection identifies cases with more evidence of true infection. As with any disease, clinical judgment should always be used along with the results of diagnostic tests. No test is ever completely accurate, so it may be reasonable on clinical grounds to treat a patient for CDI if the CCTA or even the CC (or proxy tests for these reference assays) is negative.

COMMERCIAL *CLOSTRIDIUM DIFFICILE* TESTS

There are multiple commercial tests for *C difficile*, which broadly detect 3 different targets. Toxin immunoassays (both membrane and toxEIAs) detect free toxin, as in the CCTA. Glutamate dehydrogenase (GDH) tests and NAATs detect the presence of all and toxigenic *C difficile* strains, respectively, and are summarized in **Table 1**.

Much the same reasoning used in the discussion on the association of *C difficile* reference tests with CDI also applies to commercial assays. It is important to make 3 general points about their assessment. First, commercial assays should always be tested against the appropriate gold-standard reference test, to ensure there is a comparison of like with like (in terms of which *C difficile* target is sought). For example, if a toxEIA is compared with CC as a reference test, it will detect far fewer positives and so will appear to have falsely low sensitivity. Second, estimates of diagnostic accuracy, such as sensitivity or specificity, are relatively imprecise unless the studies are large. Studies with several hundred to a few thousand specimens are required to estimate sensitivity with 95% confidence intervals less than 5% to 10%. Third, as CDI prevalence decreases, the positive predictive value (PPV) of a test result also decreases, because most samples assayed will not be from individuals with CDI; however, the

Table 1
Summary of available commercial tests for CDI

Test	Sensitivity	Specificity	Availability	Cost (US$)[a]	Substance Detected
CC	High	Low	Limited	10–20	Toxigenic *C difficile* vegetative cells or spores
CCTA	High	High	Limited	5–15	Free toxins
GDH	High	Low	Wide	5–15	Common *C difficile* enzyme antigen
Toxin immunoassays	Low	Moderate	Wide	5–15	Free toxins
NAATs	High	Low/moderate	Wide	30–50	Toxigenic *C difficile*

Abbreviations: CC, cytotoxigenic culture; CCTA, cell cytotoxin assay; GDH, glutamate dehydrogenase; NAATs, nucleic acid amplification tests.
[a] Cost of goods; does not include labor costs.

negative predictive value (NPV) will remain relatively high. A systematic review of toxEIA studies showed that these had been performed using a wide variation in CDI prevalence rates (range 6%–53%, median 15%).[52] PPVs and NPVs should be recalculated taking account of the local prevalence of disease, so as to reduce misleading interpretations of test accuracy.

There is debate about which are acceptable values for sensitivity and specificity of a test. The answer in part depends on the prevalence of CDI in the population tested[17,52]; at a prevalence of about 5% or 10%, tests should ideally have specificities of greater than 99% and sensitivities between 85% and 90%., The overall performance of diagnostic tests cannot simply be compared by comparing sensitivity or specificity of individual tests.[53] Sensitivity and specificity are inversely related. If a test has a low cutoff, it will have higher sensitivity and lower specificity than an identical test with a higher cutoff. Comparison of the performance of tests should be done with an analysis that incorporates both sensitivity and specificity, such as the comparison of area under receiver-operator characteristics curves (AUCROCC).[53]

Immunoassays

CDT and GDH immunoassays use similar technologies to detect the presence of antigens (using antibodies) in fecal samples. These tests can be performed using multiple approaches, ranging from large, automated, robotic machines (using toxEIAs) in the laboratory that can perform hundreds of tests per day, to small lateral flow and membrane capture cards (similar to commercial pregnancy tests) that may be used to rapidly detect antigen in fecal specimens. Although there are differences in performance between different immunoassays,[17,52] there is no one particular format that is better than another, and the choice of platform and format often depends on convenience for the laboratory or test setting. For example, a large laboratory testing 40 or 50 samples a day may use an automated toxEIA, whereas a membrane assay is more appropriate for rapid testing in a laboratory or even at the patient's bedside. Several manufacturers produce combined assays that detect both CDT and GDH (see later discussion).

Toxin immunoassays

For several years these inexpensive, rapid, and simple to perform assays were the commercial tests of choice for most laboratories for the diagnosis of CDI.[36,54] As some *C difficile* strains do not produce toxin A, it is recommended that toxin immunoassays should detect both toxins A and B. Feces specimens may be kept at 4°C for days or weeks before being assayed for toxin, but freeze-thawing of samples reduces the sensitivity of these tests.[55] Test sensitivities in earlier studies were reported to be 69% to 99%, with specificities of 94% to 100%,[56–64] although these were relatively small (typically <500 samples). Recent reports have claimed sensitivities of toxEIAs to be less than 60%,[65] although these studies compared EIA with CC. A more recent large study showed sensitivity of 2 toxEIAs to be 68% to 83% with specificities of approximately 99%.[12] The performance of toxin immunoassays varies markedly across manufacturers,[17] so it is important to select a relatively sensitive EIA. The overall poor performance of toxin immunoassays led to the recommendation that these should not be used as stand-alone tests, but rather as a part of a 2-stage or 3-stage algorithm.[17,52]

Glutamate dehydrogenase immunoassays

GDH immunoassays detect a highly conserved "common" antigen (enzyme) in *C difficile*.[66] As with the toxin immunoassays, these tests are relatively simple and cheap to perform. The assays detect both toxigenic and nontoxigenic *C difficile* strains and so have a low specificity (~75–92%) for CDI or versus CC,[19,58,67] although these results were from mainly small studies. A recent large study of more than 12,000 fecal samples showed that a GDH EIA had sensitivity (95% confidence interval [CI]) and specificity (95% CI) of 94.5% (92.9–95.8) and 94.5% (94.1–94.9), respectively, compared with CC, confirming this test to have high sensitivity but low specificity. For this reason GDH is only recommended to be used in combination with other assays, such as a toxin immunoassay.[68,69]

Nucleic Acid Amplification Tests

At least 9 commercial NAATs are approved by the Food and Drug Administration. These tests usually detect the *tcd A* or *tcd B* genes on the PaLoc locus; they provide a shortcut route to determining whether a strain is toxigenic, and as such are most similar to CC. NAATs are more expensive than the immunoassays, costing around $30 to $50 (excluding labor). These tests usually take about 1 to 2 hours to give a result, with most commercial assays allowing small batches or individual samples to be examined, although some commercial platforms are suitable for testing large sample numbers. In comparison with CC, NAATs have sensitivities of 70% to 100% and specificities of 94% to 100%[56,60,65,70,71]; again, however, these data come from relatively small studies, and so the lower 95% CI estimates for specificity are between 70% and 85%. A large multicenter study found sensitivity (95% CI) of 93.2% (90.8–95.1) and specificity of 96.9% (96.5–97.4) when compared with CC.[12] As would be expected, specificities were much lower when the NAAT was compared with CCTA (as the former does not detect free toxin).

Consequently, although they yield more positive results the specificities of NAATs, and thus the PPVs, are probably too low for these to be used as stand-alone tests. It has been argued that a stand-alone NAAT can be used to help diagnose CDI quickly, and for positive samples a clinical review and decision made regarding whether to treat.[72] However, given the difficulty in clinically distinguishing CDI from the many other causes of diarrhea, reported PPVs for NAATs as low as 54% (in comparison with CCTA) mean that relying on these assays alone to detect CDI has clear disadvantages. More specifically, NAATs yield about 50% to 80% more positives than CCTA,[12,49] so their use alone is likely to lead to overdiagnosis of CDI, overtreatment, and excessive use of isolation resources. NAATs are no better than CC in predicting disease, with NAAT-positive/CCTA-negative cases having indistinguishable severity markers and death rates compared with negative controls.[12]

TEST PERFORMANCE VARIATION

There is great variation between studies in the reported performance characteristics of *C difficile* tests; for example, reported sensitivity estimates for the same commercial assay (Meridian Premier) vary between 67%[12] and 99%.[62] Some of this variation may be explained by small studies with large CIs for estimates of sensitivity and specificity. Variations in the way reference tests or the commercial assays are performed may also explain differences between test estimates. However, variations in test performance have been seen in multicenter trials, despite good internal quality assurance of testing procedures.[12] These differences in test performance may result from patient selection; for example, greater numbers of patients with nontoxigenic strains may alter the reported specificities of a GDH EIA. Factors relating to the organism itself may alter the diagnostic performance of these diagnostic assays. The test performances of GDH EIAs have been reported to vary according to *C difficile* ribotype,[73] although

other studies have not confirmed this association.[74] It is possible that as yet unidentified human-related or microbe-related factors can affect test performance.

OTHER TESTS

Several other testing methodologies have been tried for diagnosing CDI, although
none can be recommended for routine use at present. Some tests have been designed
to identify patients with severe CDI. Lactoferrin and calprotectin are neutrophil-
derived fecal biomarkers of colonic inflammation that have been used extensively in
the management of inflammatory bowel disease.[75] The use of these biomarkers is
not appropriate for diagnosing CDI, owing to a very low specificity.[76] Fecal lactoferrin
has been shown to be higher in severe CDI,[77,78] but its role in individual patient management is yet to be confirmed; it is not possible at present to base changes in patient
management on a positive or negative fecal lactoferrin assay.

COMBINATIONS OF TESTS

As no commercial assays appear to have the requisite performance characteristics to
be used as stand-alone tests, combining available assays may be a way of improving
the diagnosis of CDI. The combination of more than 1 test into a testing algorithm is usual
in virology for the diagnosis of hepatitis B or human immunodeficiency virus (HIV), but it
is less common in bacteriology. The attraction of using an algorithm is that it offers a simple solution for improved diagnosis without having to wait for the development of new
diagnostic methodology. The idea of performing 2-step or 3-step laboratory algorithms
to improve CDI diagnosis has been proposed since at least 2006.[79,80]

There are several possible methods of combining assays.

- Tests may be performed in series, with a second test performed if the first test is
  positive; for example, confirmation of a positive HIV test. Most 2-step algorithms
  suggested for diagnosing CDI rely on this strategy.
- Tests may be performed in series, with a second test performed if the first test is
  negative; for example, when confirming the absence of rubella antibodies in
  pregnancy.
- Tests may be performed in parallel. These results are usually combined in a
  single result, such as fourth-generation HIV tests for HIV antibody and GP24.

The performance of the first 2-step strategy can be predicted with the following
equations:

$$\text{Algorithm\_specificity} = \text{spec}_{test1} + (\text{spec}_{test2} \times (1 - \text{spec}_{test1}))$$

$$\text{Algorithm\_sensitivity} = \text{sens}_{test1} \times \text{sens}_{test2}$$

It can be seen from these formulae that such test combinations have an overall increase in specificity with an associated decrease in sensitivity. The only exception to
this would be performing a reference assay, which by definition has a sensitivity of
100%. Manufacturers' cutoffs are nearly always used to define positive and negative
results, although these are optimized for their use in single-stage assays. It may be
possible to improve diagnostic accuracy by using a different set of cutoffs, but this
would require either manufacturer or independent validations.

There have been relatively few robust studies comparing 2-stage or 3-stage algorithms with single assays; many cannot be fully interpreted because they do not
include the use of reference tests,[50,79] or have incomplete analysis, including

comparing sensitivity rather than overall performance,[65] which as noted earlier will always be reduced in a 2-stage algorithm. A large study compared the results of 2-stage algorithms with individual tests, using more than 12,000 fecal samples. A GDH EIA, 2 toxin EIAs, and a NAAT were compared with both CC and CCTA. The best performing algorithms were then compared in the testing set.[12] Assay performances of 2-stage algorithms, as reflected in AUCROCC, were significantly higher than those for individual tests. This finding demonstrates the advantage of 2-stage algorithms over individual NAAT, toxin EIA, or GDH EIAs. The best performing algorithms are shown in **Table 2**. It should be noted that, despite the improved performance compared with individual tests, the best 2-stage algorithm to predict CC had 92% sensitivity but specificity of 98%. The best 2-stage algorithm for the prediction of CCTA had 82% sensitivity but specificity of 99.6%. There is therefore still a need to improve the performance of *C difficile* tests to optimize their specificity relative to CC and their sensitivity compared with CCTA.

WHEN AND WHO TO TEST

The selection of who to test for CDI is critically important. As there is such a high rate of CC-positive fecal samples in asymptomatic patients, it is important to test samples only in patients with diarrhea (with the very rare exception of patients with severe colitis who may have no diarrhea). There is, however, a tension in defining what is meant by diarrhea. There is a need to detect CDI as quickly as possible, both to treat patients and for infection control purposes; it can be argued, therefore, that a fecal sample should be examined for CDI after the first episode of loose stool. However, given the high frequency of loose stools, to improve the PPV of testing it is suggested that fecal samples are tested for CDI only after 3 loose stools (in a 24-hour period). This strategy may lead to delays in diagnosis from several hours to days, but has the advantage of only testing patients more likely to have CDI. Testing early will likely improve treatment and infection control outcomes, whereas testing later will improve diagnostic accuracy in terms of PPV. This tension is reflected by differences in guidelines; for example, in England it is recommended to test fecal samples for CDI after 1 unformed stool,[81] whereas guidance in the United States endorses testing only patients with 3 or more unformed stools in a 24-hour period.[68]

There is great variation between and within countries in the frequency of CDI testing. For example, in 2008 there was a 47-fold variance across European countries (3 vs 141 tests performed per 10,000 patient days) in the rate of CDI testing in hospitals.[20] The rates of CDI were higher when testing was more frequent, implying that cases of CDI are missed because of undertesting. A survey of Spanish laboratory diagnosis received all unformed fecal samples sent to routine diagnostic laboratories in Spain on a single day.[82] The study received about 75% of all samples sent to Spanish laboratories on that day. When compared with the *C difficile* test results, the routine diagnostic laboratories underestimated the number of cases of CDI by about 25%,

| Table 2 | | |
| Best performing 2-stage algorithms | | |
Reference Test	Best Performing Algorithm	Comments
CCTA	NAAT + CDT EIA	GDH EIA + CDT EIA nearly identical. Statistically not different
CC	GDH EIA + NAAT	

Abbreviation: CDT, *C difficile* toxin.

primarily because of undertesting (ie, physicians not requesting the test). A large pan-European study performed in almost 500 hospitals in 20 countries in 2013 has estimated that there are approximately 40,000 missed CDI diagnoses per year.[83]

Variability in rates of *C difficile* testing between institutions may in part be due to differences in the prevalence of hospital diarrhea. However, the major driver seems to be whether testing occurs by default (ie, on all unformed stool samples sent to the laboratory regardless of the tests requested) or only occurs on physician request. In the United Kingdom,[81] Ireland, and some other European countries, all unformed fecal samples received by the laboratory are tested for *C difficile*. Given that there is a tendency for individual physicians to underconsider CDI and thus underrequest *C difficile* testing, there is a strong argument on the grounds of control of infection and patient safety to test all unformed fecal samples sent to a laboratory for evidence of CDI.

TESTING STRATEGY

For the aforestated reasons, there should be a decision as to whether to only test on physician request, with the inherent risks of underdetection, or to test all unformed samples sent to the laboratory. Testing formed samples is unhelpful. Test selection will depend on the facilities and time available, and on the reason for testing. In essence, the detection of free toxin with CCTA or equivalent tests indicates that the patient has diarrhea caused by *C difficile*. Detection of toxigenic *C difficile* indicates that the patient represents a risk for spreading *C difficile* to other patients (and may have CDI). The tests selected should depend on which question(s) is (are) being asked. Reference tests take several days, which is usually too long for patient management; this means that CCTA and CC are usually used in research for epidemiologic or validation studies. For most diagnostic laboratories, same-day commercial assays are likely to be most appropriate.

Given the improved diagnostic performance when commercial assays are being used, 2-stage (or 3-stage) algorithms thus have advantages. If the purpose of testing

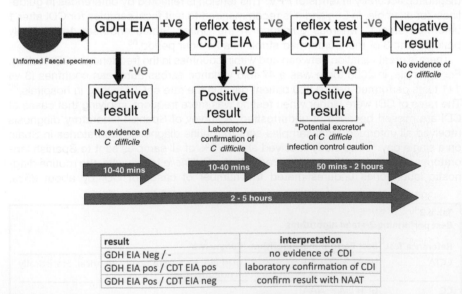

Fig. 6. Two-stage or 3-stage algorithm for the detection of CDI. CDT, *C difficile* toxin; EIA, enzyme immunoassay; GDH, glutamate dehydrogenase.

is to find toxigenic *C difficile* (and so reproduce the results of CC), performing a screening assay with a GDH EIA followed by a NAAT is appropriate. As around 80% to 90% of the samples will be negative and the GDH assays are considerably cheaper than NAAT, this is likely to be a cost-effective strategy. GDH EIAs take less than an hour to perform and so there is no long overall delay, with reports still being possible within 2 to 3 hours.

If the purpose of testing is to find free toxin (and so reproduce the results of CCTA), a 2-stage test with an initial sensitive screening test (GDH EIA or NAAT), followed by confirmation of the presence of toxin with a toxEIA, is appropriate. It is then a straight-forward task to interpret specimens that are GDH EIA negative and those that are GDH EIA positive/toxEIA positive. However, samples that have discordant results (ie, GDH EIA positive and toxEIA negative) present a potential difficulty. About half of these discordant samples are CC positive, so further testing is needed if identification of which of these patients are 'potential excretors' of *C difficile* is considered necessary. A third stage (eg, with a NAAT) can also be performed (**Fig. 6**). This 3-stage algorithm has the advantage of enabling a laboratory to, in effect, reflect the results of both refer-ence assays but produce same-day results.

SUMMARY

The diagnosis of CDI is not straightforward. Awareness of the array of available testing alternatives, how these are affected by who is tested, and when this is carried out is important, so that hospitals can select a strategy that best fits clinical need. When devising a diagnostic strategy, there needs to be clarity about the questions to be answered and the resources and time available. Two-stage testing improves diag-nostic performance of all commercial assays, although even the best algorithms do not have 100% diagnostic accuracy for CDI. Laboratory diagnostics play a key role in CDI detection and management decisions, but results should always be interpreted in the context of the clinical picture.

REFERENCES

1. Elliott B, Chang BJ, Golledge CL, et al. *Clostridium difficile*-associated diarrhoea. Intern Med J 2007;37(8):561–8.
2. Rupnik M, Wilcox MH, Gerding DN. *Clostridium difficile* infection: new develop-ments in epidemiology and pathogenesis. Nat Rev Microbiol 2009;7(7):526–36.
3. Cohen SH, Tang YJ, Silva J Jr. Analysis of the pathogenicity locus in *Clostridium difficile* strains. J Infect Dis 2000;181(2):659–63.
4. Voth DE, Ballard JD. *Clostridium difficile* toxins: mechanism of action and role in disease. Clin Microbiol Rev 2005;18(2):247–63.
5. Kyne L, Warny M, Qamar A, et al. Asymptomatic carriage of *Clostridium difficile* and serum levels of IgG antibody against toxin A. N Engl J Med 2000;342(6): 390–7.
6. Kelly CP, Kyne L. The host immune response to *Clostridium difficile*. J Med Micro-biol 2011;60(Pt 8):1070–9.
7. Klevens RM, Edwards JR, Richards CL Jr, et al. Estimating health care-associated infections and deaths in U.S. hospitals, 2002. Public Health Rep 2007;122(2):160–6.
8. Loo VG, Poirier L, Miller MA, et al. A predominantly clonal multi-institutional outbreak of *Clostridium difficile*-associated diarrhea with high morbidity and mor-tality. N Engl J Med 2005;353(23):2442–9.

9. Pepin J, Valiquette L, Gagnon S, et al. Outcomes of *Clostridium difficile*-associated disease treated with metronidazole or vancomycin before and after the emergence of NAP1/027. Am J Gastroenterol 2007;102(12):2781–8.

10. Pepin J, Valiquette L, Cossette B. Mortality attributable to nosocomial *Clostridium difficile*-associated disease during an epidemic caused by a hypervirulent strain in Quebec. CMAJ 2005;173(9):1037–42.

11. Pepin J, Valiquette L, Alary ME, et al. *Clostridium difficile*-associated diarrhea in a region of Quebec from 1991 to 2003: a changing pattern of disease severity. CMAJ 2004;171(5):466–72.

12. Planche TD, Davies KA, Coen PG, et al. Differences in outcome according to *Clostridium difficile* testing method: a prospective multicentre diagnostic validation study of *C. difficile* infection. Lancet Infect Dis 2013;13:936–45.

13. Dallal RM, Harbrecht BG, Boujoukas AJ, et al. Fulminant *Clostridium difficile*: an underappreciated and increasing cause of death and complications. Ann Surg 2002;235(3):363–72.

14. Wilson V, Cheek L, Satta G, et al. Predictors of death after *Clostridium difficile* infection: a report on 128 strain-typed cases from a teaching hospital in the United Kingdom. Clin Infect Dis 2010;50(12):e77–81.

15. Garey KW, Graham G, Gerard L, et al. Prevalence of diarrhea at a university hospital and association with modifiable risk factors. Ann Pharmacother 2006;40(6):1030–4.

16. DiPersio JR, Varga FJ, Conwell DL, et al. Development of a rapid enzyme immunoassay for *Clostridium difficile* toxin A and its use in the diagnosis of *C. difficile*-associated disease. J Clin Microbiol 1991;29(12):2724–30.

17. Eastwood K, Else P, Charlett A, et al. Comparison of nine commercially available *Clostridium difficile* toxin detection assays, a real-time PCR assay for *C. difficile* tcdB, and a glutamate dehydrogenase detection assay to cytotoxin testing and cytotoxigenic culture methods. J Clin Microbiol 2009;47(10):3211–7.

18. Fedorko DP, Engler HD, O'Shaughnessy EM, et al. Evaluation of two rapid assays for detection of *Clostridium difficile* toxin A in stool specimens. J Clin Microbiol 1999;37(9):3044–7.

19. Vanpoucke H, De Baere T, Claeys G, et al. Evaluation of six commercial assays for the rapid detection of *Clostridium difficile* toxin and/or antigen in stool specimens. Clin Microbiol Infect 2001;7(2):55–64.

20. Bauer MP, Notermans DW, van Benthem BH, et al, ECDIS Study Group. *Clostridium difficile* infection in Europe: a hospital-based survey. Lancet 2011;377(9759):63–73.

21. Phillips KD, Rogers PA. Rapid detection and presumptive identification of *Clostridium difficile* by p-cresol production on a selective medium. J Clin Pathol 1981;34(6):642–4.

22. Aronsson B, Mollby R, Nord CE. Antimicrobial agents and *Clostridium difficile* in acute enteric disease: epidemiological data from Sweden, 1980-1982. J Infect Dis 1985;151(3):476–81.

23. Clabots CR, Johnson S, Olson MM, et al. Acquisition of *Clostridium difficile* by hospitalized patients: evidence for colonized new admissions as a source of infection. J Infect Dis 1992;166(3):561–7.

24. Shim JK, Johnson S, Samore MH, et al. Primary symptomless colonisation by *Clostridium difficile* and decreased risk of subsequent diarrhoea. Lancet 1998;351(9103):633–6.

25. Samore MH, DeGirolami PC, Tlucko A, et al. *Clostridium difficile* colonization and diarrhea at a tertiary care hospital. Clin Infect Dis 1994;18(2):181–7.

26. McFarland LV, Mulligan ME, Kwok RY, et al. Nosocomial acquisition of *Clostridium difficile* infection. N Engl J Med 1989;320(4):204–10.
27. Chang TW, Lauermann M, Bartlett JG. Cytotoxicity assay in antibiotic-associated colitis. J Infect Dis 1979;140(5):765–70.
28. Donta ST, Sullivan N, Wilkins TD. Differential effects of *Clostridium difficile* toxins on tissue-cultured cells. J Clin Microbiol 1982;15(6):1157–8.
29. Maniar AC, Williams TW, Hammond GW. Detection of *Clostridium difficile* toxin in various tissue culture monolayers. J Clin Microbiol 1987;25(10):1999–2000.
30. Murray PR, Weber CJ. Detection of *Clostridium difficile* cytotoxin in HEp-2 and CHO cell lines. Diagn Microbiol Infect Dis 1983;1(4):331–3.
31. Buggy BP, Wilson KH, Fekety R. Comparison of methods for recovery of *Clostridium difficile* from an environmental surface. J Clin Microbiol 1983;18(2): 348–52.
32. Borriello SP, Honour P. Simplified procedure for the routine isolation of *Clostridium difficile* from faeces. J Clin Pathol 1981;34(10):1124–7.
33. Peterson LR, Olson MM, Shanholtzer CJ, et al. Results of a prospective, 18-month clinical evaluation of culture, cytotoxin testing, and culturette brand (CDT) latex testing in the diagnosis of *Clostridium difficile*-associated diarrhea. Diagn Microbiol Infect Dis 1988;10(2):85–91.
34. Dhawan B, Chaudhry R, Sharma N. Incidence of *Clostridium difficile* infection: a prospective study in an Indian hospital. J Hosp Infect 1999;43(4):275–80.
35. George WL, Sutter VL, Citron D, et al. Selective and differential medium for isolation of *Clostridium difficile*. J Clin Microbiol 1979;9(2):214–9.
36. Barbut F, Delmee M, Brazier JS, et al. European survey of diagnostic methods and testing protocols for *Clostridium difficile*. Clin Microbiol Infect 2003;9(10):989–96.
37. Schue V, Green GA, Monteil H. Comparison of the ToxA test with cytotoxicity assay and culture for the detection of *Clostridium difficile*-associated diarrhoea disease. J Med Microbiol 1994;41(5):316–8.
38. Merz CS, Kramer C, Forman M, et al. Comparison of four commercially available rapid enzyme immunoassays with cytotoxin assay for detection of *Clostridium difficile* toxin(s) from stool specimens. J Clin Microbiol 1994;32(5):1142–7.
39. Kelly MT, Champagne SG, Sherlock CH, et al. Commercial latex agglutination test for detection of *Clostridium difficile*-associated diarrhea. J Clin Microbiol 1987; 25(7):1244–7.
40. Wilcox MH, Eastwood KA. CEP08054: evaluation report *Clostridium difficile* toxin detection assays. London: Centre for Evidence-Based Purchasing; 2009.
41. Barbut F, Braun M, Burghoffer B, et al. Rapid detection of toxigenic strains of *Clostridium difficile* in diarrheal stools by real-time PCR. J Clin Microbiol 2009, 47(4):1276–7.
42. Sloan LM, Duresko BJ, Gustafson DR, et al. Comparison of real-time PCR for detection of the tcdC gene with four toxin immunoassays and culture in diagnosis of *Clostridium difficile* infection. J Clin Microbiol 2008;46(6):1996–2001.
43. Gerding DN, Olson MM, Peterson LR, et al. *Clostridium difficile*-associated diarrhea and colitis in adults. A prospective case-controlled epidemiologic study. Arch Intern Med 1986;146(1):95–100.
44. George WL, Rolfe RD, Harding GK, et al. *Clostridium difficile* and cytotoxin in feces of patients with antimicrobial agent-associated pseudomembranous colitis. Infection 1982;10(4):205–8.
45. George WL, Rolfe RD, Finegold SM. *Clostridium difficile* and its cytotoxin in feces of patients with antimicrobial agent-associated diarrhea and miscellaneous conditions. J Clin Microbiol 1982;15(6):1049–53.

46. Lashner BA, Todorczuk J, Sahm DF, et al. *Clostridium difficile* culture-positive toxin-negative diarrhea. Am J Gastroenterol 1986;81(10):940–3.
47. White HD, Chew DP. Acute myocardial infarction. Lancet 2008;372(9638):570–84.
48. Fox KA, Steg PG, Eagle KA, et al. Decline in rates of death and heart failure in acute coronary syndromes, 1999–2006. JAMA 2007;297(17):1892–900.
49. Longtin Y, Trottier S, Brochu G, et al. Impact of the type of diagnostic assay on *Clostridium difficile* infection and complication rates in a mandatory reporting program. Clin Infect Dis 2013;56(1):67–73.
50. Orendi JM, Monnery DJ, Manzoor S, et al. A two-stage algorithm for *Clostridium difficile* including PCR: can we replace the toxin EIA? J Hosp Infect 2012;80(1):82–4.
51. Baker I, Leeming JP, Reynolds R, et al. Clinical relevance of a positive molecular test in the diagnosis of *Clostridium difficile* infection. J Hosp Infect 2013;84(4):311–5.
52. Planche T, Aghaizu A, Holliman R, et al. Diagnosis of *Clostridium difficile* infection by toxin detection kits: a systematic review. Lancet Infect Dis 2008;8:777–84.
53. Pepe MS. The statistical evaluation of medical tests for classification and prediction. 1st edition. Oxford Statistical Science Series. Oxford (United Kingdom): Oxford University Press; 2003. p. 320.
54. Goldenberg SD, French GL. Diagnostic testing for *Clostridium difficile*: a comprehensive survey of laboratories in England. J Hosp Infect 2011;79(1):4–7.
55. Freeman J, Wilcox MH. The effects of storage conditions on viability of *Clostridium difficile* vegetative cells and spores and toxin activity in human faeces. J Clin Pathol 2003;56(2):126–8.
56. van den Berg RJ, Vaessen N, Endtz HP, et al. Evaluation of real-time PCR and conventional diagnostic methods for the detection of *Clostridium difficile*-associated diarrhoea in a prospective multicentre study. J Med Microbiol 2007;56(Pt 1):36–42.
57. Snell H, Ramos M, Longo S, et al. Performance of the TechLab C. DIFF CHEK-60 enzyme immunoassay (EIA) in combination with the *C. difficile* Tox A/B II EIA kit, the Triage *C. difficile* panel immunoassay, and a cytotoxin assay for diagnosis of *Clostridium difficile*-associated diarrhea. J Clin Microbiol 2004;42(10):4863–5.
58. Massey V, Gregson DB, Chagla AH, et al. Clinical usefulness of components of the Triage immunoassay, enzyme immunoassay for toxins A and B, and cytotoxin B tissue culture assay for the diagnosis of *Clostridium difficile* diarrhea. Am J Clin Pathol 2003;119(1):45–9.
59. O'Connor D, Hynes P, Cormican M, et al. Evaluation of methods for detection of toxins in specimens of feces submitted for diagnosis of *Clostridium difficile*-associated diarrhea. J Clin Microbiol 2001;39(8):2846–9.
60. van den Berg RJ, Bruijnesteijn van Coppenraet LS, Gerritsen HJ, et al. Prospective multicenter evaluation of a new immunoassay and real-time PCR for rapid diagnosis of *Clostridium difficile*-associated diarrhea in hospitalized patients. J Clin Microbiol 2005;43(10):5338–40.
61. Leeming J, Ferguson J, Kulpoo D, et al. Comparison of methods of *Clostridium difficile* toxins. Clin Microbiol Infect 2006;12(Suppl 4):P1643.
62. Musher DM, Manhas A, Jain P, et al. Detection of *Clostridium difficile* toxin: comparison of enzyme immunoassay results with results obtained by cytotoxicity assay. J Clin Microbiol 2007;45(8):2737–9.
63. Reyes RC, John MA, Ayotte DL, et al. Performance of TechLab C. DIFF QUIK CHEK and TechLab *C. difficile* TOX A/B II for the detection of *Clostridium difficile* in stool samples. Diagn Microbiol Infect Dis 2007;59(1):33–7.

64. Russmann H, Panthel K, Bader RC, et al. Evaluation of three rapid assays for detection of *Clostridium difficile* toxin A and toxin B in stool specimens. Eur J Clin Microbiol Infect Dis 2007;26(2):115–9.

65. Novak-Weekley SM, Marlowe EM, Miller JM, et al. *Clostridium difficile* testing in the clinical laboratory by use of multiple testing algorithms. J Clin Microbiol 2010;48(3):889–93.

66. Carman RJ, Wickham KN, Chen L, et al. Glutamate dehydrogenase is highly conserved among *Clostridium difficile* ribotypes. J Clin Microbiol 2012;50(4):1425–6.

67. Turgeon DK, Novicki TJ, Quick J, et al. Six rapid tests for direct detection of *Clostridium difficile* and its toxins in fecal samples compared with the fibroblast cytotoxicity assay. J Clin Microbiol 2003;41(2):667–70.

68. Cohen SH, Gerding DN, Johnson S, et al, Society for Healthcare Epidemiology of America, Infectious Diseases Society of America. Clinical practice guidelines for *Clostridium difficile* infection in adults: 2010 update by the Society for Healthcare Epidemiology of America (SHEA) and the Infectious Diseases Society of America (IDSA). Infect Control Hosp Epidemiol 2010;31(5):431–55.

69. Crobach MJ, Dekkers OM, Wilcox MH, et al. European Society of Clinical Microbiology and Infectious Diseases (ESCMID): data review and recommendations for diagnosing *Clostridium difficile*-infection (CDI). Clin Microbiol Infect 2009; 15(12):1053–66.

70. Stamper PD, Alcabasa R, Aird D, et al. Comparison of a commercial real-time PCR assay for tcdB detection to a cell culture cytotoxicity assay and toxigenic culture for direct detection of toxin-producing *Clostridium difficile* in clinical samples. J Clin Microbiol 2009;47(2):373–8.

71. Larson AM, Fung AM, Fang FC. Evaluation of tcdB real-time PCR in a three-step diagnostic algorithm for detection of toxigenic *Clostridium difficile*. J Clin Microbiol 2010;48(1):124–30.

72. Wilcox MH, Planche T, Fang FC, et al. Point-counterpoint. What is the current role of algorithmic approaches for diagnosis of *Clostridium difficile* infection? J Clin Microbiol 2010;48(12):4347–53.

73. Tenover FC, Novak-Weekley S, Woods CW, et al. Impact of strain type on detection of toxigenic *Clostridium difficile*: comparison of molecular diagnostic and enzyme immunoassay approaches. J Clin Microbiol 2010;48(10):3719–24.

74. Goldenberg SD, Gumban M, Hall A, et al. Lack of effect of strain type on detection of toxigenic *Clostridium difficile* by glutamate dehydrogenase and polymerase chain reaction. Diagn Microbiol Infect Dis 2011;70(3):417–9.

75. Abraham BP, Kane S. Fecal markers: calprotectin and lactoferrin. Gastroenterol Clin North Am 2012;41(2):483–95.

76. Whitehead SJ, Shipman KE, Cooper M, et al. Is there any value in measuring faecal calprotectin in *Clostridium difficile* positive faecal samples? J Med Microbiol 2014;63(Pt 4):590–3.

77. Boone JH, Archbald-Pannone LR, Wickham KN, et al. Ribotype 027 *Clostridium difficile* infections with measurable stool toxin have increased lactoferrin and are associated with a higher mortality. Eur J Clin Microbiol Infect Dis 2014;33(6): 1045–51.

78. El Feghaly RE, Stauber JL, Deych E, et al. Markers of intestinal inflammation, not bacterial burden, correlate with clinical outcomes in *Clostridium difficile* infection. Clin Infect Dis 2013;56(12):1713–21.

79. Ticehurst JR, Aird DZ, Dam LM, et al. Effective detection of toxigenic *Clostridium difficile* by a two-step algorithm including tests for antigen and cytotoxin. J Clin Microbiol 2006;44(3):1145–9.

80. Fenner L, Widmer AF, Goy G, et al. Rapid and reliable diagnostic algorithm for detection of *Clostridium difficile*. J Clin Microbiol 2008;46(1):328–30.

81. Health Protection Agency (HPA), Department of Health. *Clostridium difficile* infection: how to deal with the problem. London: Department of Health; 2008.

82. Alcala L, Martin A, Marin M, et al. *Clostridium difficile* Study, The undiagnosed cases of *Clostridium difficile* infection in a whole nation: where is the problem? Clin Microbiol Infect 2012;18(7):E204–13.

83. Davies KA, Longshaw CM, Davis GL, et al. Underdiagnosis of Clostridium difficile across Europe: the European, multicentre, prospective, biannual, point-prevalence study of Clostridium difficile infection in hospitalised patients with diarrhoea (EUCLID). Lancet Infect Dis 2014;14(12):1208–19.

Environmental Interventions to Control *Clostridium difficile*

Vivian G. Loo, MD, MSc

KEYWORDS

- *Clostridium difficile* • Infection control and prevention • Hand hygiene
- Isolation measures • Environmental disinfection

KEY POINTS

- *Clostridium difficile* is a spore-forming bacterium that can survive in the environment for several months.
- Health care workers must use contact precautions that include wearing gloves and gowns when entering the room of a patient with *C difficile* infection (CDI).
- Contact precautions should be continued for the duration of diarrhea.
- Patients with CDI should be accommodated in a private room.
- Single-use equipment should be used when possible. Reusable equipment must be cleaned and disinfected effectively.
- Chlorine-based agents are the most effective agents for environmental disinfection.

INTRODUCTION

Clostridium difficile is recognized to be the leading cause of health care–associated diarrhea. Since 2000, there has been a dramatic increase in the incidence *C difficile* infection (CDI) with associated morbidity and mortality. Most of these outbreaks have been associated with the emergence of a hypervirulent *C difficile* strain, known as the North American PFGE type 1 (NAP1) or ribotype 027.[1,2]

The ways patients may be exposed to *C difficile* in the hospital setting include (1) contact with the contaminated environment, (2) contact with a health care worker with transient hand colonization, or (3) direct contact with a patient with CDI. The rate of acquisition during hospitalization increases linearly with time and can be as high as 40% after 4 weeks of hospitalization.[3] *C difficile* forms spores and poses challenges for its control. There may not be a single method that is effective in minimizing exposure to *C difficile* and a multifaceted approach is usually required.[4–7] Different

Departments of Medicine and Microbiology, McGill University Health Centre, 687 Pine Avenue West, Room L5.06, Montreal, Quebec H3A 1A1, Canada
E-mail address: vivian.loo@muhc.mcgill.ca

Infect Dis Clin N Am 29 (2015) 83–91
http://dx.doi.org/10.1016/j.idc.2014.11.006
0891-5520/15/$ – see front matter © 2015 Elsevier Inc. All rights reserved.

id.theclinics.com

methods may be more or less effective in different institutions, depending on the local epidemiology and the available resources. This article focuses on the hospital infection control and prevention strategies against CDI.

HAND HYGIENE

Transmission of C difficile strains commonly occurs via the hands of health care workers. After caring for patients with CDI, the proportion of health care workers with hand contamination ranges from 14% to 59%.[8–11] Hand hygiene is considered to be one of the cornerstones of prevention of transmission of C difficile, as it is for most other health care–associated infections. Several studies have documented the reduction of health care–associated infections by improvement in the compliance with hand washing by health care workers after patient contact.[12] However, many studies have also documented low rates of hand washing by health care workers.[12,13] The introduction of alcohol-based hand antiseptics has been considered transformative for improving hand hygiene compliance.[12] Hand hygiene guidelines promote the use of alcohol-based products, unless the hands have come into contact with body fluids or are visibly soiled.[14] These alcohol-based antiseptics are popular because of their effectiveness in reducing hand carriage of most vegetative bacteria and many viruses, and their ease of use at the point of care. However, C difficile, in its spore form, is known to be highly resistant to killing by alcohol. Indeed, the addition of ethanol to stool samples in the laboratory facilitates the recovery of C difficile from these specimens.[15] Therefore, health care workers who decontaminate their hands with alcohol-based products may simply displace spores over the skin surface, rather than physically removing C difficile spores by mechanical washing with soap and water. This could potentially increase the risk of transferring C difficile to patients in their care. However, several studies have not demonstrated an association between the use of alcohol-based hand hygiene products and increased incidence of CDI. Gordin[16] assessed the impact of using an alcohol-based hand hygiene product on rates of infection with methicillin-resistant Staphylococcus aureus, vancomycin-resistant Enterococcus, and CDI 3 years before and after implementation. After implementation, a 21% reduction was observed in the rate of methicillin-resistant S aureus infection, and a 41% decrease in the rate of vancomycin-resistant Enterococcus infection.[16] The incidence of CDI was essentially unchanged and did not increase with the implementation of the alcohol-based hand hygiene product.[16] This finding is consistent and has been reproduced in several other studies.[17–20] Several studies have compared the use of alcohol-based products with other methods of hand hygiene.[21,22] These studies assessed the efficacy of different hand washing methods among volunteers for removal of a nontoxigenic strain of C difficile. These studies demonstrated that hand washing with soap and water, or with an antimicrobial soap and water, to be more effective at removing C difficile spores than alcohol-based hand hygiene products.[21,22] McFarland and colleagues[8] suggested that antiseptic containing chlorhexidine was more effective than plain soap for removing C difficile from the hands of health care workers. They found that C difficile persisted on the hands of 88% of personnel (14 of 16) who had washed with plain soap. Washing with 4% chlorhexidine gluconate reduced the rate to 14% (1 of 7 personnel).[8] Another study involving experimental hand seeding with C difficile showed no difference between plain soap and chlorhexidine gluconate in removing C difficile from hands.[23]

In summary, there is a theoretic potential for alcohol-based hand hygiene products to increase the incidence of CDI because of their relative ineffectiveness at eliminating spores from the hands. However, there have not been any clinical studies to support that the use of alcohol-based hand hygiene products results in an increased incidence of CDI. Hence, the Society for Healthcare Epidemiology of America–Infectious Diseases Society of America (SHEA-IDSA) Clinical Practice Guidelines for CDI recommend the preferential use of soap and water for hand hygiene over alcohol-based hand hygiene products only in CDI outbreak settings and to use alcohol-based hand hygiene products in nonoutbreak settings.[24]

PATIENT HAND HYGIENE AND BATHING

The hands of patients can also become contaminated with *C difficile*. A recent study found that 9 out of 28 (32%) patients with CDI and 6 out of 16 (38%) asymptomatic carriers had positive hand cultures before performing hand hygiene.[25] Potentially, these patients can act as vectors of transmission and this could be a factor in CDI recurrence when the spores are ingested from their hands. Theoretically, patient bathing could also decrease skin contamination of *C difficile*. Among 37 subjects with CDI, showering was more effective than bed bathing in decreasing the rate of positive skin cultures.[26] Encouraging patients to wash hands and shower could be a useful strategy to reduce the burden of spores on the skin.

CONTACT PRECAUTIONS

The use of additional isolation techniques (contact precautions, private rooms, and cohorting of patients with active CDI) has been used for control of outbreaks with varied success.[7,27,28] Contact precautions include the donning of gowns and gloves when caring for patients with CDI. There is much evidence for the contamination of health care workers' hands with *C difficile* spores, particularly when gloves are not used.[8] The use of gloves in conjunction with hand hygiene should decrease the concentration of *C difficile* organisms on the hands of health care personnel. A prospective controlled trial of vinyl glove use for handling body substances showed a significant decline in CDI rates, from 7.7 cases per 1000 discharges to 1.5 cases per 1000 discharges, before and after institution of glove use ($P = .015$), respectively.[29] After removal of gloves worn during the care of patients with CDI, it is important to practice hand hygiene. The use of gowns has been recommended because of potential soiling and contamination of the uniforms of health care personnel with *C difficile*. *C difficile* has been detected on nursing uniforms; however, a study found no evidence of the uniforms being a source of transmission to patients.[30]

It is important to place patients suspected of having CDI on contact precautions before confirmation by test results. In a prospective study of 100 subjects suspected of CDI, skin contamination was evaluated as well as the average time from placement of test orders to availability of test results. The potential for health care worker hand contamination was assessed by using sterile gloves after contact with frequently examined subject skin sites and then the gloves were imprinted onto agar for *C difficile* culture. Twenty of these 100 subjects (20%) were found to be positive for CDI and test results were available in 2.07 days. The frequency of acquisition of *C difficile* on gloved hands after skin contact with these subjects was high at 69%.[31] This study lends support that patients with suspected CDI should be placed on preemptive contact precautions pending the *C difficile* test results.

The CDC currently recommends that contact precautions be continued for the duration of the illness.[24] United Kingdom guidelines recommend continuing contact precautions for at least 48 hours after diarrhea resolves.[32] In a prospective study of 52 subjects, *C difficile* was suppressed to undetectable levels in stool samples from most subjects during treatment.[33] However, at the time of resolution of diarrhea, skin and environmental contamination were high at 60% and 37%, respectively.[33] However, data do not exist to support extending the contact precautions as a routine measure to decrease CDI incidence. Therefore, prolonging contact precautions until discharge remains a special control measure if CDI rates remain high despite implementation of standard infection control measures against CDI.[24]

ROOM ACCOMMODATION

Room design and access to hand washing facilities are important factors in the control of CDI. In a cohort study of health care–associated acquisition of CDI, there were higher acquisition rates in double rooms than in single rooms (17% vs 7%; $P = .08$) and a significantly higher risk of acquisition after exposure to a roommate with a positive culture result. In addition, it has been shown that exposure to hospital roommates is associated with an 11% increased risk of acquiring CDI; being in a private room provided protection against CDI acquisition. The effect of private rooms on CDI and other bacterial acquisition rates was studied when an intensive care unit was converted to only private rooms with easily accessible hand washing facilities.[34] A significant reduction in CDI rates by 43% was demonstrated although other confounders such as antibiotic use were not studied.[34] In a study of 1770 subjects admitted to the intensive care unit and housed in rooms whose previous occupants did not have CDI, 4.6% developed CDI. For those who were placed in rooms whose previous occupants did have CDI, 11.0% developed CDI.[35] The previous occupant's CDI status remained a significant risk factor for CDI development when adjusted for other potential confounding variables such as age, comorbidity, antibiotic, and proton pump inhibitor use. This study illustrates the importance of environmental disinfection to prevent transmission.

Cohorting patients with CDI in a multibed room may occur because private rooms may not be available. The risk of recurrence was studied among subjects with CDI admitted to a cohort ward and adjusted for potential risk factors such as age, continued antibiotic use, and comorbidities.[36] Admission to a *C difficile* cohort ward was found to be an independent predictor for recurrence.[36] If cohorting is necessary, dedicated commodes should be provided to patients to avoid further cross-contamination.

In conclusion, patients with CDI should be placed in a private room to decrease transmission to other patients and rooms must be effectively cleaned and disinfected.

ENVIRONMENTAL CLEANING AND DISINFECTION

The surface environment in rooms housing patients with CDI is frequently contaminated with *C difficile*. *C difficile* has been cultured from various surfaces including floors, commodes, toilets, bed pans, call bells, and overbed tables.[8,10] *C difficile* spores can survive in the environment for months or years due to their innate resistance to drying, heat, and certain disinfectants.[37,38] Notably, epidemic *C difficile* strains may have a greater sporulation capacity in vitro than do nonoutbreak strains.[38] Studies have found that the rate of environmental contamination by *C difficile* increases according to the carriage and symptom status of the subjects. It was lowest in rooms of culture-negative subjects (fewer than 8% of environmental surfaces), intermediate in rooms of subjects with asymptomatic *C difficile* colonization (8%–30% of environmental surfaces), and highest in rooms of subjects with CDI (9%–50% of environmental surfaces).[8,37] Samore[10] showed that the environmental prevalence of *C difficile* correlated with the extent of contamination of health care workers' hands by this bacterium. For example, hand contamination was 0%, 8%, and 26% when environmental contamination was 0% to 25%, 26% to 50%, and greater than 50%, respectively.

Hypochlorite-based disinfectants are recommended for disinfection of environmental surfaces in rooms of patients with CDI because they are sporicidal at 1000 ppm. There are several reports that using chlorine-based agents can reduce environmental contamination by C difficile and an associated decrease in CDI incidence.[39,40] Introduction of cleaning with a hypochlorite-based solution (5000 ppm available chlorine) was associated with reduced incidence of CDI in a bone marrow transplant unit where there was a relatively high infection rate.[39] The incidence of CDI increased almost to the baseline level after the reintroduction of the original quaternary ammonium compound as the principal cleaning agent. However, the environmental prevalence of C difficile contamination was not measured in this study, and the results were not reproducible with patients on other units, possibly because of the low prevalence of infection. Wilcox[41] used a crossover study design to demonstrate a significant correlation between the use of a cleaning agent containing 1000 ppm available chlorine and a reduction in the incidence of CDI on 1 of the 2 hospital wards that were examined. Daily disinfection of high-touch surfaces will also decrease the environmental contamination with C difficile. Daily cleaning along with disinfection with sodium hypochlorite, compared with disinfection of these surfaces only when visibly soiled, decreased environmental contamination and hand contamination of health care workers.[42] This is another strategy to prevent cross-transmission.

Chlorine-based products are not effective in removing organic material. Mechanical cleaning with a germicide is required before the use of hypochlorite-based agents to lower the spore burden by physical removal.[43] Moreover, hypochlorite-based disinfectants are limited by their corrosive nature on metal surfaces. Although it is likely that higher concentrations of available chlorine within the range of 1000 to 5000 ppm are more reliably sporicidal than lower concentrations, practical issues may limit the use of such products for routine cleaning (eg, causticity to surfaces, complaints from personnel about the odor, and possible hypersensitivity).[43] Therefore, depending on such factors, the concentration of available chlorine should be at least 1000 ppm and may ideally be 5000 ppm. It is important to follow the manufacturer's recommendations for the surface contact time of the disinfectant.

Quaternary ammonium solutions are commonly used disinfectants in the hospital setting in some countries. In vitro exposure of epidemic C difficile strains, including NAP1/BI/027, to subinhibitory concentrations of nonchlorine-based cleaning agents (detergent or hydrogen peroxide) significantly increased sporulation capacity; this effect was not seen with chlorine-based cleaning agents.[44] These results suggest the possibility that some cleaning agents, if allowed to come into contact with C difficile in low concentrations, could promote sporulation and, therefore, enhance the persistence of the bacterium in the environment.[44]

Recent reports have highlighted the use of no-touch methods such as ultraviolet light or hydrogen peroxide vapor to further reduce the level of environmental contamination by C difficile.[45-49] These studies found that both HPV and ultraviolet light further reduced environmental contamination by C difficile after surfaces have already been disinfected with hypochlorite agents. However, the attributable impact on CDI incidence was difficult to establish because other measures were instituted concomitantly. In addition, there are practical limitations with HPV, such as the need to vacate and seal rooms and to have access to specialized equipment. Similarly, with ultraviolet light, there is a need to vacate the room, special equipment is required, and the items to be decontaminated must be in the line of sight of the device.

The thoroughness of cleaning is important. Each health care facility should have a standard operating procedure to clean and disinfect surfaces. It is reported that up to 50% of hospital surfaces are not cleaned appropriately by environmental staff during terminal cleaning.[50] Barriers to effective cleaning may be due insufficient time for cleaning, inadequate cleaning supplies, inadequate education, and poor communication.[51] Direct observation with real-time feedback, fluorescent markers, and adenosine triphosphate bioluminescence are valuable tools to improve cleaning practices.[49,52,53]

MEDICAL EQUIPMENT

Single-use disposable equipment should be used for prevention of CDI transmission. Nondisposable medical equipment should be dedicated to the patient's room, and other equipment should be thoroughly cleaned after use in a patient with CDI. Environmental contamination has been linked to the spread of C difficile by way of contaminated commodes, blood pressure cuffs, and oral and rectal thermometers.[8,54,55] Replacement of electronic thermometers with single-use disposable thermometers has been associated with significant reductions in CDI incidence.[56] In a recent study, stethoscopes were found to acquire and transfer C difficile spores as often as gloved hands during simulated routine physical examinations on subjects with CDI.[57] These results support the recommendation to use disposable patient equipment when possible and to ensure that reusable equipment is well cleaned and disinfected.

SUMMARY

The control of CDI is of great importance. Hand hygiene, isolation measures, and environmental disinfection are important factors to decrease CDI incidence. An infection control bundle strategy is often required to successfully control CDI outbreaks.[7,58] These interventions are multifaceted and include health care worker education, rapid case finding, enhanced environmental cleaning with chlorine-based disinfectants, contact precautions, private room accommodation of patients with CDI, hand washing with soap and water, and antimicrobial stewardship.

REFERENCES

1. McDonald LC, Lessa F, Sievert D, et al. Vital signs: preventing Clostridium difficile infections. MMWR Morb Mortal Wkly Rep 2012;61(9):157–62.
2. Loo VG, Poirier L, Miller M, et al. A predominantly clonal multi-institutional outbreak of Clostridium difficile-associated diarrhea with high morbidity and mortality. N Engl J Med 2005;353:2442–9.
3. Clabots CR. Acquisition of Clostridium difficile by hospitalized patients: evidence for colonized new admissions as a source of infection. J Infect Dis 1992;166:561–7.
4. Apisarnthanarak A. Effectiveness of environmental and infection control programs to reduce transmission of Clostridium difficile. Clin Infect Dis 2004;39:601–2.
5. Cartmill TD. Management and control of a large outbreak of diarrhoea due to Clostridium difficile. J Hosp Infect 1994;27:1–15.
6. Stone SP. The effect of an enhanced infection-control policy on the incidence of Clostridium difficile infection and methicillin-resistant Staphylococcus aureus colonization in acute elderly medical patients. Age Ageing 1998;27:561–8.

7. Muto CA, Blank K, Marsh J, et al. Control of an outbreak of infection with the hypervirulent *Clostridium difficile* BI strain in a university hospital using a comprehensive "bundle" approach. Clin Infect Dis 2007;45(10):1266–73.
8. McFarland LV, Mulligan ME, Kwok R, et al. Nosocomial acquisition of *Clostridium difficile* infection. N Engl J Med 1989;320(4):203–10.
9. Landelle C, Verachten M, Legrand P, et al. Contamination of healthcare workers' hands with *Clostridium difficile* spores after caring for patients with *C difficile* infection. Infect Control Hosp Epidemiol 2014;35(1):10–5.
10. Samore MH. Clinical and molecular epidemiology of sporadic and clustered cases of nosocomial *Clostridium difficile* diarrhea. Am J Med 1996;100:32–40.
11. Guerrero DM, Nerandzic MM, Jury LA, et al. Acquisition of spores on gloved hands after contact with the skin of patients with *Clostridium difficile* infection and with environmental surfaces in their rooms. Am J Infect Control 2012;40(6):556–8.
12. Boyce JM. Using alcohol for hand antisepsis: dispelling old myths. Infect Control Hosp Epidemiol 2000;21(7):438–41.
13. Pittet D, Mourouga P, Perneger TV. Compliance with handwashing in a teaching hospital. Infection Control Program. Ann Intern Med 1999;130(2):126–30.
14. World Health Organization. WHO Guidelines on Hand Hygiene in Health Care. 2009. Available at: http://whqlibdoc.who.int/publications/2009/9789241597906_eng.pdf?ua=1. Accessed July 18, 2014.
15. Clabots CR, Gerding SJ, Olson MM, et al. Detection of asymptomatic *Clostridium difficile* carriage by an alcohol shock procedure. J Clin Microbiol 1989;27(10):2386–7.
16. Gordin FM. Reduction in nosocomial transmission of drug-resistant bacteria after introduction of an alcohol-based handrub. Infect Control Hosp Epidemiol 2005;26:650–3.
17. Boyce JM. Lack of association between the increased incidence of *Clostridium difficile* - associated disease and the increasing use of alcohol-based hand rubs. Infect Control Hosp Epidemiol 2006;27:479–83.
18. Kaier K, Hagist C, Frank U, et al. Two time-series analyses of the impact of antibiotic consumption and alcohol-based hand disinfection on the incidences of nosocomial methicillin-resistant *Staphylococcus aureus* infection and *Clostridium difficile* infection. Infect Control Hosp Epidemiol 2009;30(4):346–53.
19. Knight N, Strait T, Anthony N, et al. *Clostridium difficile* colitis: a retrospective study of incidence and severity before and after institution of an alcohol-based hand rub policy. Am J Infect Control 2010;38(7):523–8.
20. Vernaz N, Sax H, Pittet D, et al. Temporal effects of antibiotic use and hand rub consumption on the incidence of MRSA and *Clostridium difficile*. J Antimicrob Chemother 2008;62(3):601–7.
21. Oughton MT, Loo VG, Dendukuri N, et al. Hand hygiene with soap and water is superior to alcohol rub and antiseptic wipes for removal of *Clostridium difficile*. Infect Control Hosp Epidemiol 2009;30(10):939–44.
22. Jabbar U, Leischner J, Kasper D, et al. Effectiveness of alcohol-based hand rubs for removal of *Clostridium difficile* spores from hands. Infect Control Hosp Epidemiol 2010;31(6):565–70.
23. Bettin KM. Effectiveness of liquid soap vs chlorhexidine gluconate for the removal of *Clostridium difficile* from bare hands and gloved hands. Infect Control Hosp Epidemiol 1994;15(11):697–702.
24. Dubberke ER, Carling PM, Carrico RP, et al. Strategies to prevent clostridium difficile infections in acute care hospitals: 2014 update. Infect Control Hosp Epidemiol 2014;35(6):628–45.

25. Kundrapu S, Sunkesula V, Jury I, et al. A randomized trial of soap and water hand wash versus alcohol hand rub for removal of *Clostridium difficile* spores from hands of patients. Infect Control Hosp Epidemiol 2014;35(2):204–6.

26. Jury LA, Guerrero DM, Burant CJ, et al. Effectiveness of routine patient bathing to decrease the burden of spores on the skin of patients with *Clostridium difficile* infection. Infect Control Hosp Epidemiol 2011;32(2):181–4.

27. Cartmill TD. Nosocomial diarrhoea due to a single strain of *Clostridium difficile*: a prolonged outbreak in elderly patients. Age Ageing 1992;21:245–9.

28. Salgado CD, Mauldin PD, Fogle PJ, et al. Analysis of an outbreak of *Clostridium difficile* infection controlled with enhanced infection control measures. Am J Infect Control 2009;37(6):458–64.

29. Johnson S. Prospective, controlled study of vinyl glove use to interrupt *Clostridium difficile* nosocomial transmission. Am J Med 1990;88:137–40.

30. Perry C. Bacteria contamination of uniforms. J Hosp Infect 2001;48:238–41.

31. Sunkesula VC, Kundrapu S, Jury LA, et al. Potential for transmission of spores by patients awaiting laboratory testing to confirm suspected *Clostridium difficile* infection. Infect Control Hosp Epidemiol 2013;34(3):306–8.

32. Department of Health. *Clostridium difficile* infection: how to deal with the problem. London: Department of Health; 2008. Available at: http://www.hpa.org.uk/webc/HPAwebFile/HPAweb_C/1232006607827.

33. Sethi AK, Al-Nassir WN, Nerandzic MM, et al. Persistence of skin contamination and environmental shedding of *Clostridium difficile* during and after treatment of *C difficile* infection. Infect Control Hosp Epidemiol 2010;31(1):21–7.

34. Teltsch DY, Hanley J, Loo VG, et al. Infection acquisition following intensive care unit room privatization. Arch Intern Med 2011;171(1):32–8.

35. Shaughnessy MK, Micielli RL, DePestel DD, et al. Evaluation of hospital room assignment and acquisition of *Clostridium difficile* infection. Infect Control Hosp Epidemiol 2011;32(3):201–6.

36. Islam J, Cheek E, Navani V, et al. Influence of cohorting patients with *Clostridium difficile* infection on risk of symptomatic recurrence. J Hosp Infect 2013;85(1):17–21.

37. Kim KH, Fekety R, Batts DH, et al. Isolation of *Clostridium difficile* from the environment and contacts of patients with antibiotic-associated colitis. J Infect Dis 1981;143(1):42–50.

38. Fawley WN, Underwood S, Freeman J, et al. Efficacy of hospital cleaning agents and germicides against epidemic *Clostridium difficile* strains. Infect Control Hosp Epidemiol 2007;28(8):920–5.

39. Mayfield JL, Leet T, Miller J, et al. Environmental control to reduce transmission of *Clostridium difficile*. Clin Infect Dis 2000;31:995–1000.

40. Hacek D, Ogle AM, Fisher A, et al. Significant impact of terminal room cleaning with bleach on reducing nosocomial *Clostridium difficile*. Am J Infect Control 2010;38:350–3.

41. Wilcox MH. Comparison of the effect of detergent versus hypochlorite cleaning on environmental contamination and incidence of *Clostridium difficile* infection. J Hosp Infect 2003;54:109–14.

42. Kundrapu S, Sunkesula V, Jury LA, et al. Daily disinfection of high-touch surfaces in isolation rooms to reduce contamination of healthcare workers' hands. Infect Control Hosp Epidemiol 2012;33(10):1039–42.

43. Rutala WA, Weber DJ. Uses of inorganic hypochlorite (bleach) in health-care facilities. Clin Microbiol Rev 1997;10(4):597–610.

44. Wilcox MH. Hospital disinfectants and spore formation by *Clostridium difficile*. Lancet 2006;356:1324.

45. Best EL, Parnell P, Thirkell G, et al. Effectiveness of deep cleaning followed by hydrogen peroxide decontamination during high *Clostridium difficile* infection incidence. J Hosp Infect 2014;87(1):25–33.
46. Manian FA, Griesnauer S, Bryant A. Implementation of hospital-wide enhanced terminal cleaning of targeted patient rooms and its impact on endemic *Clostridium difficile* infection rates. Am J Infect Control 2013;41:537–41.
47. Passaretti CL, Otter JA, Reich NG, et al. An evaluation of environmental decontamination with hydrogen peroxide vapor for reducing the risk of patient acquisition of multidrug-resistant organisms. Clin Infect Dis 2013;56(1):27–35.
48. Boyce JM, Havill NL, Otter JA, et al. Impact of hydrogen peroxide vapor room decontamination on *Clostridium difficile* environmental contamination and transmission in a healthcare setting. Infect Control Hosp Epidemiol 2008;29(8):723–9.
49. Sitzlar BB, Deshpande AM, Fertelli D, et al. An environmental disinfection odyssey: evaluation of sequential interventions to improve disinfection of clostridium difficile isolation rooms. Infect Control Hosp Epidemiol 2013;34(5):459–65.
50. Carling PC, Parry MM, Rupp ME, et al. Improving cleaning of the environment surrounding patients in 36 acute care hospitals. Infect Control Hosp Epidemiol 2008; 29(11):1035–41.
51. Jennings A, Sitzlar B, Jury L. A survey of environmental service workers' knowledge and opinions regarding environmental cleaning. Am J Infect Control 2013;41(2):177–9.
52. Guerrero DM, Carling PC, Jury LA, et al. Beyond the Hawthorne effect: reduction of clostridium difficile environmental contamination through active intervention to improve cleaning practices. Infect Control Hosp Epidemiol 2013;34(5):524–6.
53. Deshpande A, Sitzlar B, Fertelli D, et al. Utility of an adenosine triphosphate bioluminescence assay to evaluate disinfection of *Clostridium difficile* isolation rooms. Infect Control Hosp Epidemiol 2013;34(8):865–7.
54. Manian FA, Meyer L, Jenne J. *Clostridium difficile* contamination of blood pressure cuffs: a call for a closer look at gloving practices in the era on universal precautions. Infect Control Hosp Epidemiol 1996;17(3):180–2.
55. Brooks S, Khan A, Stoica D, et al. Reduction in vancomycin-resistant *Enterococcus* and *Clostridium difficile* infections following change to tympanic thermometers. Infect Control Hosp Epidemiol 1998;19(5):333–6.
56. Jernigan JA. A randomized crossover study of disposable thermometers for prevention of *Clostridium difficile* and other nosocomial infections. Infect Control Hosp Epidemiol 1998;19:494–9.
57. Vajravelu RK, Guerrero DM, Jury LA, et al. Evaluation of stethoscopes as vectors of *Clostridium difficile* and methicillin-resistant *Staphylococcus aureus*. Infect Control Hosp Epidemiol 2012;33(1):96–8.
58. Weiss K, Boisvert A, Chagnon M, et al. Multipronged intervention strategy to control an outbreak of *Clostridium difficile* infection (CDI) and its impact on the rates of CDI from 2002 to 2007. Infect Control Hosp Epidemiol 2009;30(2):156–62.

Treatment of *Clostridium difficile* Infections

Melinda M. Soriano, PharmD[a], Stuart Johnson, MD[b],*

KEYWORDS

- *Clostridium difficile* • Antibiotic • Treatment

KEY POINTS

- Two recent, randomized, controlled studies have helped define the role of vancomycin and fidaxomicin in the treatment of *Clostridium difficile* infections (CDI).
- The first study confirmed higher cure rates using vancomycin over metronidazole for patients with an initial or recurrent CDI episode.
- The second study confirmed superior sustained response for fidaxomicin over vancomycin for patients with an initial or first CDI recurrence.
- In patients with multiple recurrent CDI, nonstandard antibiotic treatments, including taper and pulse strategy, using vancomycin and potentially, fidaxomicin may be effective.

INTRODUCTION

Since the recognition of the disease in the mid to late 1970s, treatment of *Clostridium difficile* infections (CDI) has undergone several changes both in routine clinical practice and in the recommendations of guideline committees. Vancomycin was the first agent shown to be effective in the treatment of pseudomembranous colitis; treatment of pseudomembranous colitis with vancomycin was established before *C difficile* was confirmed as the etiology.[1] This agent remains a highly effective treatment for CDI to this day. Vancomycin achieves high fecal concentrations when given orally, and clinically important resistance to this agent among *C difficile* isolates has never been reported.

Despite reservations about its pharmacokinetic profile, metronidazole was also studied and shown to be effective in the treatment of CDI. Primarily because of its lower cost and apparent similar efficacy to vancomycin, metronidazole treatment of CDI increased through the 1980s, and in the 1990s it became the preferred treatment for many clinicians and authorities.[2] In 1995, the US Centers for Disease Control and Prevention recommended that the use of vancomycin in hospitals be reduced out of

a Department of Pharmacy, Presence Resurrection Medical Center, 7435 West Talcott Avenue, Chicago, IL 60631, USA; b Research Service, Hines VA Hospital, 5000 South 5th Street, Hines, IL 60141, USA
* Corresponding author.
E-mail address: stuart.johnson2@va.gov

Infect Dis Clin N Am 29 (2015) 93–108
http://dx.doi.org/10.1016/j.idc.2014.11.005
0891-5520/15/$ – see front matter Published by Elsevier Inc.

concern for emergence of vancomycin resistance in other pathogens.[3] Also in 1995, the Society for Healthcare Epidemiology published a Position Paper on *C difficile*-associated diarrhea and colitis.[4] This paper recommended 10 days of treatment with either vancomycin or metronidazole as effective, but suggested that metronidazole may be preferred.

Subsequently, there have been increasing reports of slow clinical response times and decreased microbiological responses to treatment with metronidazole.[5,6] In 2007, a randomized trial of metronidazole and vancomycin reported similar efficacy for mild CDI, but decreased efficacy of metronidazole for treatment in patients with severe CDI.[7] The updated CDI guidelines from Society for Healthcare Epidemiology and the Infectious Diseases Society of America published in 2010 recommended vancomycin as the drug of choice for severe disease and recommended treatment with either agent for mild-to-moderate CDI. Although both agents were studied as 10-day regimens, a 10- to 14-day course was recommended primarily because of data showing a slow response to metronidazole.[8] The definition of severe CDI is not yet universally agreed upon, but with the understanding that metronidazole is highly absorbed and that only modest drug levels are achieved in the stool during active infection, there is decreasing enthusiasm for this agent, particularly in patients with severe CDI. The results of the large, international, multicenter, placebo-controlled trial of vancomycin, metronidazole, and tolevamer have further defined the relative efficacy of metronidazole in CDI.[9] This study represents the largest and arguably the most rigorous comparative trial of these agents and showed that vancomycin was superior in efficacy to metronidazole overall, regardless of disease severity. Tolevamer is an investigational drug that, after its disappointing results in this trial, is unlikely to become available.[9]

This review discusses new outcome measures for comparing CDI treatments; agents available for treatment, including the newly approved agent, fidaxomicin; and considerations for modifying therapy in patients with severe, complicated CDI and recurrent CDI.

EVALUATION OF OUTCOMES

Symptomatic response while on therapy is the first and most important treatment outcome and has been used to compare all proposed agents for CDI. Most trials have compared 10-day regimens and there are data to suggest that treatment durations of less than 10 days result in lower cure rates.[10] Despite high initial cure rates, particularly with vancomycin, recurrence of symptoms after discontinuation of treatment is frequent and has led investigators to use sustained response as an alternative treatment outcome measure.[11-13] Sustained response, previously called "global response," has been defined as resolution of symptoms during treatment without recurrence of symptoms 1 month after treatment completion. This outcome was used to distinguish important differences between vancomycin and fidaxomicin.[14] Whereas both agents gave similar, high initial cure rates, recurrent diarrhea was seen almost twice as frequently in the 1-month follow-up period with vancomycin. These results translated into a superior sustained response rate for fidaxomicin compared with vancomycin. Although sustained response was an important outcome in comparing fidaxomicin with vancomycin, this outcome could be misleading if used to compare an agent that was inferior for initial cure, but associated with lower rates of recurrence; for example, comparison of the toxin binding agent tolevamer, with metronidazole.[9] Both outcomes, initial cure and sustained response, will be important for future comparisons of CDI treatment agents.

PHARMACOLOGIC TREATMENT OPTIONS
Vancomycin

Vancomycin is a glycopeptide antibiotic that is bactericidal for all Gram-positive bacteria with the exception of enterococci.[15] It is a cell wall active agent that binds to the D-ala-D-ala precursor, which inhibits transglycosylase and subsequent peptidoglycan synthesis. Additional activity of vancomycin has been previously described and possibly includes targeting cell membrane permeability and RNA synthesis.[15,16] When given orally, the antibiotic demonstrates minimal systemic bioavailability, although rare cases of oral absorption have been described in patients with renal dysfunction and increased bowel inflammation.[17,18]

Because vancomycin has minimal oral absorption, high fecal concentrations are achieved relative to the minimum inhibitory concentration (MIC) of *C difficile* during and after treatment.[19,20] Vancomycin given at doses of 125 mg 4 times daily achieves fecal concentrations ranging between 200 and 2000 μg/mL throughout treatment.[1,20,21] The supratherapeutic concentrations of orally administered vancomycin achieved at the site of infection exceed the reported MIC for *C difficile*, with MIC_{90} ranges between 1 and 2 μg/mL.[22] Intracolonic concentrations also exceed the MIC of vancomycin for organisms with elevated MICs of 16 μg/mL.[23,24]

Oral vancomycin is approved at a dosage of 125 mg 4 times daily (**Table 1**) and this regimen was found to be as effective as vancomycin 500 mg 4 times daily in an earlier study, with comparable response rates and cessation of diarrhea in patients with probable or proven *C difficile* colitis.[25,26] A more recent retrospective study identified that vancomycin dosages totaling 500 mg/d versus more than 500 mg/d did not influence clinical cure in a multivariate model adjusted for baseline characteristics.[27] In a prospective, randomized study, Zar and colleagues[7] determined a difference in cure rates among patients meeting criteria for severe disease who received vancomycin 125 mg 4 times daily compared with oral metronidazole 250 mg 4 times daily (97% vs 76%, respectively). Vancomycin dosages of 500 mg 4 times daily are recommended in clinical guidelines for patients with severe, complicated CDI (see Severe and/or Complicated Disease); however, data supporting doses over 125 mg are not available.[2,8,28–30]

Fidaxomicin

Fidaxomicin is a macrocyclic antibiotic that is the newest antimicrobial approved for *C difficile*-associated diarrhea. It inhibits RNA synthesis by targeting DNA strand separation within RNA polymerase.[31] Fidaxomicin has limited systemic bioavailability and achieves high fecal concentrations in excess of 1000 μg/g of the parent compound and its active metabolite, OP-1118.[32] Evaluation of fecal specimens obtained from patients enrolled in phase II studies demonstrated the protective effect of fidaxomicin against reducing *Bacteroidetes* group and other commensal colonic microbiota, when compared with oral vancomycin therapy for CDI.[33,34] Additionally, fidaxomicin was found to have a longer postantibiotic effect (12.5 hours) compared with vancomycin (0–3 hours) and metronidazole (0–3 hours), and was found to inhibit both toxin production and spore production.[35–37]

Fidaxomicin was approved at a dosage of 200 mg given twice daily.[38] Two phase III studies evaluated the efficacy of fidaxomicin compared with oral vancomycin 125 mg 4 times daily for the outcomes of cure, recurrence, and the composite outcome of global cure (sustained response).[12,13] Noninferiority between the therapies was met in both trials; the rates of clinical cure were 87.7% to 88.2% for fidaxomicin and 85.8% to 86.8% for vancomycin. Recurrence rates were lower among fidaxomicin-treated patients, and translated to significantly greater sustained response rates

Table 1
Available pharmacologic treatment options

Drug (Brand)[a]	FDA Indication	Oral Dosing	Mechanism of Action	Suggested Role in CDI Therapy
Vancomycin, oral (Vancocin®)[26]	Treatment of C difficile-associated diarrhea	Adults: 125 mg orally 4 times daily for 10 d Pediatric: 40 mg/kg in 3–4 divided doses daily for 7–10 d	Inhibition of cell wall biosynthesis, bacterial–cell membrane permeability, and RNA synthesis	Initial CDI, recurrent CDI
Fidaxomicin (Dificid®)[38]	Treatment of C difficile-associated diarrhea	200 mg orally twice daily for 10 d	Inhibition of RNA polymerase [Venugopal]	Initial CDI, recurrent CDI
Metronidazole (Flagyl®)[67]	Treatment of infections owing to susceptible anaerobic bacteria	Adults: 250–750 mg 3 times daily Pediatric: 35–50 mg/kg in 3 divided doses daily	Prodrug that forms an anionic nitro radical that interacts with bacterial DNA, leading to cell death	Initial CDI (mild disease), adjunctive therapy in patients with severe ileus
Rifaximin (Xifaxan®)[58]	Treatment of patients with traveler's diarrhea owing to Escherichia coli Reduction of hepatic encephalopathy recurrence	Patients ≥12 y with traveler's diarrhea: 200 mg orally 3 times daily Patients ≥18 y with hepatic encephalopathy: 550 mg orally twice daily	Inhibits DNA-dependent RNA polymerase necessary for bacterial RNA synthesis	Postvancomycin, 'chaser' strategy for multiple recurrent CDI
Nitazoxanide (Alinia®)[68]	Diarrhea owing to Giardia lamblia or Cryptosporidium parvum	The following doses are to be taken with food: Age 1–3 y: 100 mg every 12 h Age 4–11 y: 200 mg every 12 h Age ≥12 y: 500 mg every 12 h	Inhibits pyruvate-ferredoxin oxidoreductase to inhibit anaerobic energy metabolism	Alternate therapy for initial CDI or for metronidazole failures

Abbreviation: CDI, C difficile infection.

[a] Other agents that have been studied include fusidic acid (not available in the United States, resistance concerns); bacitracin (poorly tolerated, resistance concerns); teicoplanin (not available in the United States); tigecycline (anecdotal reports of use as adjunctive therapy for severe CDI with ileus).

among fidaxomicin-treated patients compared with vancomycin-treated patients. The benefit of fidaxomicin was investigated further among subgroups of patients within the phase III trials.[39] A possible protective effect of fidaxomicin against recurrence was observed among patients with active cancers (solid or hematologic malignancy), advanced age, patients taking concomitant antibiotics, and among patients with no or mild renal failure.[40–43]

Resistance to fidaxomicin has not been reported and isolates collected from phase III studies showed MIC_{90} of 0.25 μg/mL.[44] Only 1 isolate showed an elevated MIC of 16 μg/mL and was discovered in a patient with a recurrent episode who was initially found to have a fully susceptible isolate with an MIC of 0.06 μg/mL.

Metronidazole

Metronidazole is a nitroimidazole with activity against a wide spectrum of Gram-positive and Gram-negative anaerobic organisms, including *C difficile* and *Bacteroides* spp, and protozoa. As a prodrug, metronidazole is activated by the reduction of its nitro group, creating an anionic nitro radical that interacts with bacterial DNA and leads to cell death.[45] Metronidazole has excellent oral bioavailability with almost complete absorption after an oral dose.[46] In vitro studies have demonstrated that metronidazole is bactericidal against *B fragilis* and *C perfringens* isolates, and was found to be rapidly bactericidal when compared with vancomycin.[47–49]

Although no approved dosing regimens of metronidazole for the treatment of CDI exist, a strategy of 500 mg administered 3 times daily for a 10-day course is recommended by national guidelines.[8,28] Early studies demonstrated similar efficacy between metronidazole and vancomycin and was the basis for recommendations to use metronidazole for initial CDI therapy.[2,5] Two prospective, multinational, randomized, controlled trials have evaluated tolevamer (a toxin binder) against metronidazole and vancomycin for the treatment of CDI.[9] Tolevamer was inferior to either comparator treatment for the primary endpoint of clinical success, and metronidazole was found to have a lower clinical success rate compared with vancomycin (72.7% vs 81.1%; $P = .02$). This trend of lower response to metronidazole was also consistent when evaluating clinical success according to disease severity. A post hoc logistic regression analysis using only the metronidazole and vancomycin data confirmed that vancomycin treatment was significantly associated with clinical success ($P = .034$).

Inferior outcomes with metronidazole have been attributed to subtherapeutic colonic concentrations after oral and intravenous therapy, and observed elevations in the MIC of *C difficile* isolates (although direct relationships between these and treatment failure have not been established).[50–52] Random samples obtained from patients receiving 400 to 500 mg of metronidazole 3 times daily showed fecal concentrations of 9.3, 3.3, and 1.23 μg/mL for uniformed, semiformed, and formed stool, respectively.[53] Using a Clinical and Laboratory Standards Institute MIC breakpoint of 8 μg/mL or less for susceptibility, only patients with active diarrhea achieve adequate fecal metronidazole concentrations, which possibly compromises the effectiveness of metronidazole in patients with resolving diarrhea. Rates of metronidazole resistance were found to be 7.7% in 1994, 6.3% in 2002, and 12% in 2008 among toxigenic isolates in Spain.[54–56] Reduced susceptibility was also identified among isolates from the United Kingdom obtained between 2005 and 2006, with 24% of *C difficile* ribotype 001 isolates having reduced susceptibility.[50]

Rifaximin

Rifaximin is a minimally absorbed macrolide antibiotic with broad spectrum of activity.[15] Both Gram-positive and Gram-negative aerobic and anaerobic bacteria are targeted with rifaximin; however, use of rifaximin has focused on the treatment of infections owing to methicillin-resistant Staphylococcus aureus, C difficile, and Enterobacteriaceae.[57] Rifaximin is indicated for the treatment of traveler's diarrhea owing to Escherichia coli and for preventing the recurrence of hepatic encephalopathy.[58] Dosages of 200 to 400 mg 3 times daily have been used off-label for CDI, despite the lack of an approved indication for this disease.[59,60]

Few studies have evaluated rifaximin for the treatment of initial infections owing to C difficile and a handful have looked at its utility in recurrent CDI, or CDI refractory to standard therapies.[59–63] A small, randomized trial (n = 20 patients) comparing rifaximin 200 mg 3 times daily with oral vancomycin 500 mg twice daily in patients with CDI found that rates of symptom resolution were similar.[59] In a prospective, open-label study Basu and colleagues[63] evaluated the efficacy of a 14-day course of rifaximin 400 mg 3 times daily in patients with C difficile positive stool samples after metronidzole therapy. Of the patients at the end of rifaximin therapy and at the end of a 56-day follow-up period, 64% had negative stool samples for C difficile. Rifaximin has also been evaluated as a postvancomycin "chaser" regimen in several case series and in a prospective, randomized pilot study.[60–62] After standard therapy (metronidazole or vancomycin), placebo or rifaximin 400 mg was given 3 times daily for 20 days.[60] Patients receiving rifaximin therapy reported lower rates of recurrent diarrhea (21%) compared with those receiving placebo (49%; P = .018). No difference in CDI recurrence was found between treatment groups, but the study was likely underpowered.

The ionization of rifaximin across all pH values within the gastrointestinal tract prevents oral absorption and ensures high fecal concentrations of the drug.[15] Measured fecal concentrations obtained after taking rifaximin 800 mg daily for 3 days averaged 7961 μg/g.[64] Intraluminal concentrations of rifaximin greatly exceed the MICs for most C difficile strains, but some strains demonstrate high-level resistance (range, 0.004–128 μg/mL; MIC_{90} of 128 μg/mL).[65] Like other rifamycins, development of resistance has been reported and remains a concern. The recovery of isolates found to have elevated MICs after therapy and the observed increases in resistance overall suggest caution against the routine use of rifaximin for CDI therapy.[61,62]

Nitazoxanide

Nitazoxanide is a nitrothiazolyl–salicylamide thiazolide with broad spectrum activity against both protozoa and anaerobic bacteria. It inhibits pyruvate-ferredoxin oxidoreductase and affects anaerobic energy metabolism for Helicobacter pylori, Campylobacter jejuni, anaerobic parasites and anaerobic bacteria, such as C difficile and C perfringens.[66] Nitazoxanide is approved by the US Food and Drug Administration for the treatment of diarrhea owing to Giardia lamblia and Cryptosporidium parvum with adult dosing recommended at 500 mg twice daily and appropriate dosage reductions for pediatric patients by age (see Table 1).[68] Food increases absorption of nitazoxanide. Upon absorption, nitazoxanide is deacetylated into an active metabolite, tizoxanide, and approximately two thirds of the drug is eliminated within the feces.[68,69] In vitro susceptibility testing of C difficile isolates showed MICs of nitazoxanide to range between 0.03 and 5 μg/mL, with a MIC_{90} of 0.125 μg/mL.[70]

Two prospective studies evaluated nitazoxanide for the treatment of C difficile compared with vancomycin and metronidazole, respectively.[11,71] Ten days of therapy with metronidazole 250 mg every 6 hours was compared with 7 and 10 days of nitazoxanide 500 mg every 12 hours for the primary outcome of clinical response after 7 days of therapy.[11] Clinical response at 7 days was similar between the antibiotic groups with 82.4% of metronidazole patients and 89.5% of nitazoxanide treated patients meeting the criteria for clinical response; clinical response for the 7- and 10-day nitazoxanide group was 90% and 88.9%, respectively. Sustained response at 31 days after therapy was also similar between the 3 groups. Fifty patients were randomized to receive either nitazoxanide 500 mg every 12 hours or vancomycin 125 mg every 4 hours for 10 days and were evaluated for clinical response during 3 days after therapy completion.[71] Response to therapy was similar between the groups—74% for vancomycin-treated patients and 77% for those who received nitazoxanide. In both studies, nitazoxanide efficacy was shown to be similar to that of metronidazole and vancomycin therapy for the treatment of *C difficile* infections. Nitazoxanide has also been evaluated in an open-label study for patients unresponsive to at least 14 days of metronidazole therapy or who experienced 2 recurrences within 30 days of completing therapy with either metronidazole or vancomycin.[72] Doses of nitazoxanide 500 mg every 12 hours were used and patients were followed for 60 days. Although 26 of the 35 patients evaluated experienced a response to therapy, 7 of 26 experienced a recurrence. Overall, 23 of 35 patients who received either an initial or repeated courses of nitazoxanide showed response.

Other Agents

Other agents that have been studied for treatment of CDI, but that are no longer widely used, include fusidic acid, bacitracin, teicoplanin, and tigecycline. In addition, several new therapies are being studied and may be commercially available in the near future. Two new antibacterial agents, injectable monoclonal antibodies, and a toxoid vaccine are undergoing phase III testing. A nontoxigenic *C difficile* biotherapeutic has completed phase II testing and another vaccine has just started phase II testing (**Table 2**).

SPECIAL CONSIDERATIONS FOR MODIFYING THERAPY
Severe and/or Complicated Disease

The 2010 Society for Healthcare Epidemiology/Infectious Diseases Society of America guidelines defined severe, complicated CDI as severe CDI accompanied by hypotension, shock, ileus, or megacolon.[8] The incidence of severe, complicated CDI cases increased in the early 2000s and coincided with the spread of the epidemic BI/NAP1/027 strain of *C difficile*.[73] Many of these patients do not respond to antibiotic treatment and mortality rates can be quite high. The recommended antibiotic treatment includes oral vancomycin (500 mg 4 times daily) plus intravenous metronidazole (500 mg 3 times daily) and consideration of rectal vancomycin enemas if severe ileus is present although the evidence supporting these recommendations is limited.[8] If patients do not respond to antibiotic treatment, they should be considered for operative intervention; a subtotal colectomy and end ileostomy is the procedure of choice.[74,75] Even after colectomy, 30-day mortality is around 40%.[74] Timing of surgical intervention is not well-defined, but data suggest that mortality rates are higher if the serum lactate is 5 mmol/L or higher and white blood cell count is 50,000 cells/mL or greater, or if multisystem organ failure has developed.[76,77]

Recently, a less invasive surgical option has been reported in a series of patients with severe, complicated CDI.[78] This procedure involves the creation of a diverting loop ileostomy, which can be performed laparoscopically. After creation of the ostomy, the colon is lavaged intraoperatively with a polyethylene glycol solution. After surgery, vancomycin enemas are administered in an antegrade fashion through the ostomy. Intravenous metronidazole was also administered empirically to the patients in this series. Most of the patients were eventually able to have the ileostomy reversed

Table 2
Treatment options in development

Drug (Manufacturer)	Mechanism of Action	Status of Drug Approval	Studied Dosing and Comparator	Primary Endpoint
Cadazolid (Actelion)	Inhibition of protein synthesis	Phase III	Cadazolid 250 mg orally twice daily for 10 d Oral vancomycin 125 mg 4 times daily for 10 d	Clinical cure
Surotomycin (Cubist Pharmaceuticals)	Induces rapid depolarization of bacterial cell membrane	Phase III	Surotomycin 250 mg orally twice daily for 10 d Oral vancomycin 125 mg 4 times daily for 10 d	Clinical cure
MK-6072, MK-3415A (Merck Sharpe & Dohme Corporation) ClinicalTrials.gov number NCT01513239	Human monoclonal antibody targeting *Clostridium difficile* toxin B (MK-6072), or toxins A and B (MK-3415A)	Phase III	Single infusion of: MK-6072 MK-3415A Placebo	Recurrence
VP20621 NTCD (Shire Pharmaceuticals)	Promotes colonization of NTCD	Phase II complete	10^4 NTCD for 7 d 10^7 NTCD for 7 d 10^7 NTCD for 14 d Placebo	Colonization with NTCD
H-030-012 *C difficile* toxoid vaccine (Sanofi Pasteur) ClinicalTrials.gov number NCT01887912	Stimulates production of antitoxin A and B antibodies	Phase III	1 injection of the following at days 0, 7, 30: *C difficile* toxoid vaccine Placebo	PCR confirmed primary CDI
PF-06425090 *C difficile* vaccine (Pfizer) ClinicalTrials.gov number NCT02117570	Stimulates production of antitoxin A and B antibodies	Phase II	3 doses of the following: *C difficile* vaccine Placebo	Immunogenicity Safety and tolerability

Abbreviations: CDI, *C difficile* infection; NTCD, nontoxigenic *C difficile* spores; PCR, polymerase chain reaction.

and the mortality was substantially decreased compared with their experience with colectomy (19% vs 50% historically with colectomy).[78] Although a direct comparison of this procedure with colectomy is not available, the diverting loop ileostomy may be a more attractive option to critically ill patients who might not be candidates for an open laparotomy owing to intraoperative mortality risks.

Recurrence

Among the pathophysiologic factors associated with recurrent CDI, disruption of the indigenous flora of the intestine is likely one of the most important factors. Recent data using nonculture techniques to elaborate the diversity and abundance of the fecal microbiome show a progressive loss of diversity and drop out of major bacterial groups starting with healthy patients compared with patients with initial CDI episodes, and then compared with patients with recurrent CDI.[79] With this understanding, strategies for managing recurrences in patients with initial CDI episodes or "early CDI recurrences" may not work for patients with multiple CDI recurrences in whom the fecal microbiome is markedly disrupted. This is particularly relevant for antibacterial approaches to treating recurrences. For example, despite the well-demonstrated advantage of fidaxomicin over vancomycin for decreasing the rate of subsequent recurrences, use of a standard 10-day course of fidaxomicin in patients with multiple CDI recurrences is often followed by subsequent recurrences.[80,81]

Patients with a first CDI recurrence can usually be managed with the same treatment that was used to treat the initial episode, because there is little evidence for development of resistance to agents typically used to treat CDI, particularly with regard to vancomycin.[82] However, there are concerns with regard to use of metronidazole for recurrent CDI, including reports of increased MICs of metronidazole among recent clinical *C difficile* isolates, unpredictable fecal concentrations achieved with this agent, and a risk for neurotoxicity in patients with repeated or prolonged treatment courses.[19,50,83] Comparative data for vancomycin and fidaxomicin are available for patients with a first CDI recurrence. A randomized subset of patients with first CDI recurrences was included in the multicenter, double-blinded controlled trials comparing 10-day courses of vancomycin versus fidaxomicin.[84] In this substudy, patients treated with fidaxomicin had a 20% subsequent recurrent CDI rate compared with 36% in patients treated with vancomycin ($P = .045$). These results paralleled the results seen in the overall trial, which included primarily patients with initial CDI episodes.

There are several empirical approaches to treating patients with multiple recurrences (eg, >2 CDI episodes) and these strategies can be summarized into 1 of 5 categories. With the exception of fecal microbiota transplantation and adjunctive therapy with probiotics, there are no comparative trials for any of these strategies. In addition, there is no accepted, preferable order in which to introduce these treatments. For example, a patient who had recurrences after metronidazole treatment for the first CDI episode and vancomycin treatment for the second CDI episode is now faced with several potential options for treatment of their third episode (second recurrence) and there is considerable variation among treatments offered. In general, there are some approaches to avoid, including:

- Repeated or prolonged courses of metronidazole (see rationale listed previously)
- Combination therapy (no data to support metronidazole plus vancomycin and addition of rifampin to metronidazole did not decrease recurrence rates when given for primary CDI)[85]
- Increased dosages of vancomycin (125 mg given 4 times daily achieves fecal concentrations in the mg/g range and higher dosages likely contribute to further

disruption of the indigenous flora without any beneficial effect on suppression of *C difficile*)[19]

- Concomitant antibiotics (although some concurrent conditions will dictate other antibiotic treatments, concomitant antibiotic therapy has been shown to increase risk of recurrent CDI).[9,43]

The first strategy listed for management of multiple recurrent CDI is to switch treatment agents (**Box 1**). If the patient has not previously received fidaxomicin, this agent is a logical choice, given the evidence for decreased recurrences in patients with initial and first recurrent CDI episodes. However, the number of previous CDI episodes may negatively influence the response to a standard treatment course of fidaxomicin.[81] Although not approved by the US Food and Drug Administration for CDI, nitazoxanide has shown to be helpful for some patients who have failed metronidazole therapy.[72]

Another strategy that has been used by many clinicians who treat patients with recurrent CDI is to employ taper and pulse treatment regimens. This strategy has been used primarily with vancomycin and, in this author's experience, has been effective for a majority of patients with multiple CDI recurrences. In addition, vancomycin taper and pulse regimens are often still effective if patients fail a first vancomycin taper. McFarland and colleagues[86] studied a subgroup of patients enrolled in 2 clinical trials for the probiotic *Saccharomyces*. Those patients within the placebo arm were treated for subsequent CDI episodes in a nonrandomized manner, but patients who received a vancomycin taper or a pulse regimen given once every 2 to 3 days had lower recurrence rates than patients who received a regimen of vancomycin (250 mg) given 4 times daily (31%, 14%, and 71.4%, respectively). The optimal vancomycin taper and pulse regimen is not known, but the most common regimen includes a standard 10 to 14 treatment course of 125 mg 4 times daily, followed by twice daily for a week, once daily for a week, and then once every 2 to 3 days for 2 to 8 weeks.[8] In an effort to improve response rates in patients refractory to vancomycin taper and standard 10-day fidaxomicin regimens, we have used fidaxomicin in a taper and pulsed fashion.[81] After a vancomycin taper or a 10-day fidaxomicin treatment course, 12 patients were given fidaxomicin in a 14- to 33-day tapering course (eg, 200 mg once daily for 1 week, then every other day for 3 weeks). Only 2 patients (17%) had a subsequent recurrence, and both of these patients had received concomitant antibiotics.

The third strategy listed is the postvancomycin, "chaser" regimen. We have used rifaximin, another agent not approved by the US Food and Drug Administration, as the chaser in this strategy to improve outcomes for patients who have failed multiple

---

Box 1
Strategies for managing patients with multiple recurrent *Clostridium difficile* infection episodes

- Switch treatment agent
- Taper and/or pulsed treatment regimens
- Postvancomycin chaser regimens
- Microbiota replacement approaches
- Immune approaches
- Toxin binding approaches

previous attempts to stop recurrences.[61,62] A randomized pilot study of this rifaximin chaser approach in patients with initial and recurrent CDI has also showed promise.[60] Our rationale and hypothesis for this empiric approach is that a CDI-active, "microbiota-sparing" antimicrobial (eg, rifaximin) given immediately after vancomycin therapy (used to reduce *C difficile* counts and minimize rifaximin resistance development) would allow the indigenous flora to recover and reestablish colonization resistance while *C difficile* is actively controlled. Although this approach continues to be helpful, there is concern, because isolates with high MICs of rifaximin were selected for in several patients after treatment.[61,62] Given the success with rifaximin used as a chaser, we have also empirically used fidaxomicin as a postvancomycin chaser with success.[81,87] One potential advantage of fidaxomicin over rifaximin is the lower possible risk for resistance emergence with fidaxomicin.

Microbiota replacement is a logical and direct strategy to manage patients with multiple recurrent CDI episodes. Effectiveness of fecal microbiota transplantation has now been demonstrated in a randomized trial and is covered in detail in the article by Young elsewhere in this issue.[88] Probiotics, primarily *Saccharomyces boulardii*, have also been studied as an adjunctive treatment for these patients in an attempt to instill a more healthy microbiota, but have not been convincingly effective in this setting (see the article by Allen elsewhere in this issue). It is possible that use of other, more effective probiotics or biotherapeutic agents will be effective adjunctive microbiota replacement strategies.[89]

Intravenous immunoglobulin is the only currently available immune agent for managing patients with multiple recurrences and intravenous immunoglobulin use is supported by anecdotal evidence only.[90,91] Finally, toxin-binding approaches have been advocated as a nonantibiotic approach to managing recurrent CDI, but the only available agents, cholestyramine and colestipol, have not been shown effective.[10,92] Tolevamer, a nonabsorbed polymer was shown to be ineffective for treating CDI compared with vancomycin and metronidazole, but this toxin binder or a similar agent could be resurrected and studied as adjunctive therapy.[9]

SUMMARY

The management of *C difficile* infections has evolved over the past 30 years. Antimicrobials active against *C difficile* have been the mainstay of therapy, although the emphasis has changed toward the use and development of newer agents with more narrow spectra of antibacterial activity that are less disruptive to colonic microbiota. Recurrent CDI is challenging, but most patients can be managed with currently available drugs using emerging treatment strategies. With the availability of a new agent, fidaxomicin, and the likely availability of several new therapeutic agents soon, the future for CDI management is promising.

REFERENCES

1. Tedesco F, Gurwith M, Bartlett JG, et al. Oral vancomycin for antibiotic-associated pseudomembranous colitis. Lancet 1978;2(8083):226–8.
2. Teasley DG, Gerding DN, Olson MM, et al. Prospective randomised trial of metronidazole versus vancomycin for Clostridium-difficile-associated diarrhoea and colitis. Lancet 1983;2(8358):1043–6.
3. Recommendations for preventing the spread of vancomycin resistance. Recommendations of the Hospital Infection Control Practices Advisory Committee (HICPAC). MMWR Recomm Rep 1995;44(RR–12):1–13.

4. Gerding DN, Johnson S, Peterson LR, et al. Clostridium difficile-associated diarrhea and colitis. Infect Control Hosp Epidemiol 1995;16(8):459–77.
5. Wilcox MH, Howe R. Diarrhoea caused by Clostridium difficile: response time for treatment with metronidazole and vancomycin. J Antimicrob Chemother 1995; 36(4):673–9.
6. Al-Nassir WN, Sethi AK, Nerandzic MM, et al. Comparison of clinical and microbiological response to treatment of Clostridium difficile-associated disease with metronidazole and vancomycin. Clin Infect Dis 2008;47(1):56–62.
7. Zar FA, Bakkanagari SR, Moorthi KM, et al. A comparison of vancomycin and metronidazole for the treatment of Clostridium difficile-associated diarrhea, stratified by disease severity. Clin Infect Dis 2007;45(3):302–7.
8. Cohen SH, Gerding DN, Johnson S, et al. Clinical practice guidelines for Clostridium difficile infection in adults: 2010 update by the Society for Healthcare Epidemiology of America (SHEA) and the Infectious Diseases Society of America (IDSA). Infect Control Hosp Epidemiol 2010;31(5):431–55.
9. Johnson S, Louie TJ, Gerding DN, et al. Vancomycin, metronidazole, or tolevamer for Clostridium difficile infection: results from two multinational, randomized, controlled trials. Clin Infect Dis 2014;59(3):345–54.
10. Mogg GA, Arabi Y, Youngs D, et al. Therapeutic trials of antibiotic associated colitis. Scand J Infect Dis Suppl 1980;(Suppl 22):41–5.
11. Musher DM, Logan N, Hamill RJ, et al. Nitazoxanide for the treatment of Clostridium difficile colitis. Clin Infect Dis 2006;43(4):421–7.
12. Louie TJ, Miller MA, Mullane KM, et al. Fidaxomicin versus vancomycin for Clostridium difficile infection. N Engl J Med 2011;364(5):422–31.
13. Cornely OA, Crook DW, Esposito R, et al. Fidaxomicin versus vancomycin for infection with Clostridium difficile in Europe, Canada, and the USA: a double-blind, non-inferiority, randomised controlled trial. Lancet Infect Dis 2012;12(4):281–9.
14. Johnson S, Gerding DN, Louie TJ, et al. Sustained clinical response as an endpoint in treatment trials of Clostridium difficile-associated diarrhea. Antimicrob Agents Chemother 2012;56(8):4043–5.
15. Grayson LM, Kucers A, Crowe S, et al. Kucers' The use of antibiotics sixth edition. 6th edition. London: Hodder Arnold;; 2010.
16. Jordan DC, Inniss WE. Selective inhibition of ribonucleic acid synthesis in Staphylococcus aureus by vancomycin. Nature 1959;184(Suppl 24):1894–5.
17. Aradhyula S, Manian FA, Hafidh SA, et al. Significant absorption of oral vancomycin in a patient with Clostridium difficile colitis and normal renal function. South Med J 2006;99(5):518–20.
18. Chihara S, Shimizu R, Furukata S, et al. Oral vancomycin may have significant absorption in patients with Clostridium difficile colitis. Scand J Infect Dis 2011; 43(2):149–50.
19. Johnson S, Homann SR, Bettin KM, et al. Treatment of asymptomatic Clostridium difficile carriers (fecal excretors) with vancomycin or metronidazole. A randomized, placebo-controlled trial. Ann Intern Med 1992;117(4):297–302.
20. Abujamel T, Cadnum JL, Jury LA, et al. Defining the vulnerable period for reestablishment of Clostridium difficile colonization after treatment of C. difficile infection with oral vancomycin or metronidazole. PLoS One 2013;8(10):e76269.
21. Gonzales M, Pepin J, Frost EH, et al. Faecal pharmacokinetics of orally administered vancomycin in patients with suspected Clostridium difficile infection. BMC Infect Dis 2010;10:363.
22. Pepin J. Vancomycin for the treatment of Clostridium difficile infection: for whom is this expensive bullet really magic? Clin Infect Dis 2008;46(10):1493–8.

23. Wong SS, Woo PC, Luk WK, et al. Susceptibility testing of Clostridium difficile against metronidazole and vancomycin by disk diffusion and etest. Diagn Microbiol Infect Dis 1999;34(1):1–6.

24. Aspevall O, Lundberg A, Burman LG, et al. Antimicrobial susceptibility pattern of Clostridium difficile and its relation to PCR ribotypes in a Swedish University Hospital. Antimicrob Agents Chemother 2006;50(5):1890–2.

25. Fekety R, Silva J, Kauffman C, et al. Treatment of antibiotic-associated Clostridium difficile colitis with oral vancomycin: comparison of two dosage regimens. Am J Med 1989;86(1):15–9.

26. Vancocin® [package insert]. ViroPharma Incorporated. Available at: http://www.accessdata.fda.gov/drugsatfda_docs/label/2011/050606s028lbl.pdf. Accessed September 29, 2014.

27. Lam SW, Bass SN, Neuner EA, et al. Effect of vancomycin dose on treatment outcomes in severe Clostridium difficile infection. Int J Antimicrob Agents 2013; 42(6):553–8.

28. Debast SB, Bauer MP, Kuijper EJ. European Society of Clinical Microbiology and Infectious Diseases: update of the treatment guidance document for Clostridium difficile infection. Clin Microbiol Infect 2014;20(Suppl 2):1–26.

29. Dudley MN, McLaughlin JC, Carrington G, et al. Oral bacitracin vs vancomycin therapy for Clostridium difficile-induced diarrhea. A randomized double-blind trial. Arch Intern Med 1986;146(6):1101–4.

30. de Lalla F, Nicolin R, Rinaldi E, et al. Prospective study of oral teicoplanin versus oral vancomycin for therapy of pseudomembranous colitis and Clostridium difficile-associated diarrhea. Antimicrob Agents Chemother 1992;36(10):2192–6.

31. Venugopal AA, Johnson S. Fidaxomicin: a novel macrocyclic antibiotic approved for treatment of Clostridium difficile infection. Clin Infect Dis 2012; 54(4):568–74.

32. Shue YK, Sears PS, Shangle S, et al. Safety, tolerance, and pharmacokinetic studies of opt-80 in healthy volunteers following single and multiple oral doses. Antimicrob Agents Chemother 2008;52(4):1391–5.

33. Louie TJ, Emery J, Krulicki W, et al. Opt-80 eliminates Clostridium difficile and is sparing of bacteroides species during treatment of C. difficile infection. Antimicrob Agents Chemother 2009;53(1):261–3.

34. Tannock GW, Munro K, Taylor C, et al. A new macrocyclic antibiotic, fidaxomicin (opt-80), causes less alteration to the bowel microbiota of Clostridium difficile-infected patients than does vancomycin. Microbiology (Reading, England) 2010;156(Pt 11):3354–9.

35. Babakhani F, Bouillaut L, Gomez A, et al. Fidaxomicin inhibits spore production in Clostridium difficile. Clin Infect Dis 2012,55(Suppl 2):S162–9.

36. Babakhani F, Bouillaut L, Sears P, et al. Fidaxomicin inhibits toxin production in Clostridium difficile. J Antimicrob Chemother 2013;68(3):515–22.

37. Babakhani F, Gomez A, Robert N, et al. Postantibiotic effect of fidaxomicin and its major metabolite, op-1118, against Clostridium difficile. Antimicrob Agents Chemother 2011;55(9):4427–9.

38. Dificid® [package insert]. San Diego, CA: Optimer Pharmaceuticals, Inc; 2011.

39. Soriano MM, Liao S, Danziger LH. Fidaxomicin: a minimally absorbed macrocyclic antibiotic for the treatment of Clostridium difficile infections. Expert Rev Anti Infect Ther 2013;11(8):767–76.

40. Cornely OA, Miller MA, Fantin B, et al. Resolution of Clostridium difficile-associated diarrhea in patients with cancer treated with fidaxomicin or vancomycin. J Clin Oncol 2013;31(19):2493–9.

41. Louie TJ, Miller MA, Crook DW, et al. Effect of age on treatment outcomes in Clostridium difficile infection. J Am Geriatr Soc 2013;61(2):222–30.
42. Mullane KM, Cornely OA, Crook DW, et al. Renal impairment and clinical outcomes of Clostridium difficile infection in two randomized trials. Am J Nephrol 2013;38(1):1–11.
43. Mullane KM, Miller MA, Weiss K, et al. Efficacy of fidaxomicin versus vancomycin as therapy for Clostridium difficile infection in individuals taking concomitant antibiotics for other concurrent infections. Clin Infect Dis 2011;53(5):440–7.
44. Goldstein EJ, Citron DM, Sears P, et al. Comparative susceptibilities to fidaxomicin (opt-80) of isolates collected at baseline, recurrence, and failure from patients in two phase III trials of fidaxomicin against Clostridium difficile infection. Antimicrob Agents Chemother 2011;55(11):5194–9.
45. Edwards DI. Mechanism of antimicrobial action of metronidazole. J Antimicrob Chemother 1979;5(5):499–502.
46. Lau AH, Lam NP, Piscitelli SC, et al. Clinical pharmacokinetics of metronidazole and other nitroimidazole anti-infectives. Clin Pharmacokinet 1992;23(5):328–64.
47. Ralph ED, Kirby WM. Unique bactericidal action of metronidazole against Bacteroides fragilis and Clostridium perfringens. Antimicrob Agents Chemother 1975; 8(4):409–14.
48. Stratton CW, Weeks LS, Aldridge KE. Comparison of the bactericidal activity of clindamycin and metronidazole against cefoxitin-susceptible and cefoxitin-resistant isolates of the Bacteroides fragilis group. Diagn Microbiol Infect Dis 1991;14(5):377–82.
49. Odenholt I, Walder M, Wullt M. Pharmacodynamic studies of vancomycin, metronidazole and fusidic acid against Clostridium difficile. Chemotherapy 2007;53(4): 267–74.
50. Baines SD, O'Connor R, Freeman J, et al. Emergence of reduced susceptibility to metronidazole in Clostridium difficile. J Antimicrob Chemother 2008;62(5):1046–52.
51. Brazier JS, Fawley W, Freeman J, et al. Reduced susceptibility of Clostridium difficile to metronidazole. J Antimicrob Chemother 2001;48(5):741–2.
52. Huang H, Weintraub A, Fang H, et al. Antimicrobial resistance in Clostridium difficile. Int J Antimicrob Agents 2009;34(6):516–22.
53. Bolton RP, Culshaw MA. Faecal metronidazole concentrations during oral and intravenous therapy for antibiotic associated colitis due to Clostridium difficile. Gut 1986;27(10):1169–72.
54. Pelaez T, Alcala L, Alonso R, et al. Reassessment of Clostridium difficile susceptibility to metronidazole and vancomycin. Antimicrob Agents Chemother 2002; 46(6):1647–50.
55. Pelaez T, Cercenado E, Alcala L, et al. Metronidazole resistance in Clostridium difficile is heterogeneous. J Clin Microbiol 2008;46(9):3028–32.
56. Pelaez T, Sanchez R, Blazquez R, et al. Metronidazole resistance in Clostridium difficile: a new emerging problem? Program and abstracts of the 34th Interscience Conference on Antimicrobial Agents and Chemotherapy (ICAAC). Orlando, October 4–7, 1994.
57. Scarpignato C, Pelosini I. Rifaximin, a poorly absorbed antibiotic: pharmacology and clinical potential. Chemotherapy 2005;51(Suppl 1):36–66.
58. Xifaxan® [package insert]. Salix Pharmaceuticals, Inc. Available at: http://cdn.salix.com/shared/pi/xifaxan550-pi.pdf. Accessed December 2, 2014.
59. Boero M, Berti E, Morgando A, et al. Treatment for colitis caused by Clostridium difficile: results of a randomized open study of rifaximine vs. Vancomycin. Microbiol Med (Milan) 1990;5(2):74–7.

60. Garey KW, Ghantoji SS, Shah DN, et al. A randomized, double-blind, placebo-controlled pilot study to assess the ability of rifaximin to prevent recurrent diarrhoea in patients with Clostridium difficile infection. J Antimicrob Chemother 2011;66(12):2850–5.

61. Johnson S, Schriever C, Galang M, et al. Interruption of recurrent Clostridium difficile-associated diarrhea episodes by serial therapy with vancomycin and rifaximin. Clin Infect Dis 2007;44(6):846–8.

62. Johnson S, Schriever C, Patel U, et al. Rifaximin redux: treatment of recurrent Clostridium difficile infections with rifaximin immediately post-vancomycin treatment. Anaerobe 2009;15(6):290–1.

63. Basu P, Dinani A, Rayapudi K, et al. Rifaximin therapy for metronidazole-unresponsive Clostridium difficile infection: a prospective pilot trial. Therap Adv Gastroenterol 2010;3(4):221–5.

64. Jiang ZD, Ke S, Palazzini E, et al. In vitro activity and fecal concentration of rifaximin after oral administration. Antimicrob Agents Chemother 2000;44(8):2205–6.

65. Marchese A, Salerno A, Pesce A, et al. In vitro activity of rifaximin, metronidazole and vancomycin against Clostridium difficile and the rate of selection of spontaneously resistant mutants against representative anaerobic and aerobic bacteria, including ammonia-producing species. Chemotherapy 2000;46(4): 253–66.

66. Hoffman PS, Sisson G, Croxen MA, et al. Antiparasitic drug nitazoxanide inhibits the pyruvate oxidoreductases of Helicobacter pylori, selected anaerobic bacteria and parasites, and Campylobacter jejuni. Antimicrob Agents Chemother 2007; 51(3):868–76.

67. Flagyl® [package insert]. G.D. Searle. Available at: http://labeling.pfizer.com/showlabeling.aspx?id=570. Accessed September 29, 2014.

68. Alinia® [package insert]. Romark Laboratories, L.C. Available at: http://www.romark.com/images/stories/AliniaPrescriptionInformation.pdf. Accessed September 29, 2014.

69. Broekhuysen J, Stockis A, Lins RL, et al. Nitazoxanide: pharmacokinetics and metabolism in man. Int J Clin Pharmacol Ther 2000;38(8):387–94.

70. Hecht DW, Galang MA, Sambol SP, et al. In vitro activities of 15 antimicrobial agents against 110 toxigenic Clostridium difficile clinical isolates collected from 1983 to 2004. Antimicrob Agents Chemother 2007;51(8):2716–9.

71. Musher DM, Logan N, Bressler AM, et al. Nitazoxanide versus vancomycin in Clostridium difficile infection: a randomized, double-blind study. Clin Infect Dis 2009;48(4):e41–6.

72. Musher DM, Logan N, Mehendiratta V, et al. Clostridium difficile colitis that fails conventional metronidazole therapy: response to nitazoxanide. J Antimicrob Chemother 2007;59(4):705–10.

73. Dallal RM, Harbrecht BG, Boujoukas AJ, et al. Fulminant Clostridium difficile: an underappreciated and increasing cause of death and complications. Ann Surg 2002;235(3):363–72.

74. Bhangu A, Nepogodiev D, Gupta A, et al. Systematic review and meta-analysis of outcomes following emergency surgery for Clostridium difficile colitis. Br J Surg 2012;99(11):1501–13.

75. Butala P, Divino CM. Surgical aspects of fulminant Clostridium difficile colitis. Am J Surg 2010;200(1):131–5.

76. Lamontagne F, Labbe AC, Haeck O, et al. Impact of emergency colectomy on survival of patients with fulminant Clostridium difficile colitis during an epidemic caused by a hypervirulent strain. Ann Surg 2007;245(2):267–72.

77. Perera AD, Akbari RP, Cowher MS, et al. Colectomy for fulminant Clostridium difficile colitis: predictors of mortality. Am Surg 2010;76(4):418–21.
78. Neal MD, Alverdy JC, Hall DE, et al. Diverting loop ileostomy and colonic lavage: an alternative to total abdominal colectomy for the treatment of severe, complicated Clostridium difficile associated disease. Ann Surg 2011;254(3):423–7 [discussion: 427–9].
79. Chang JY, Antonopoulos DA, Kalra A, et al. Decreased diversity of the fecal microbiome in recurrent Clostridium difficile-associated diarrhea. J Infect Dis 2008; 197(3):435–8.
80. Orenstein R. Fidaxomicin failures in recurrent Clostridium difficile infection: a problem of timing. Clin Infect Dis 2012;55(4):613–4.
81. Soriano MM, Danziger LH, Gerding DN, et al. Novel fidaxomicin treatment regimens for patients with multiple Clostridium difficile infection recurrences that are refractory to standard therapies Open Forum. Open Forum Infect Dis 2014;1(2).
82. Pepin J, Routhier S, Gagnon S, et al. Management and outcomes of a first recurrence of Clostridium difficile-associated disease in Quebec, Canada. Clin Infect Dis 2006;42(6):758–64.
83. Frytak S, Moertel CH, Childs DS. Neurologic toxicity associated with high-dose metronidazole therapy. Ann Intern Med 1978;88(3):361–2.
84. Cornely OA, Miller MA, Louie TJ, et al. Treatment of first recurrence of Clostridium difficile infection: fidaxomicin versus vancomycin. Clin Infect Dis 2012;55(Suppl 2): S154–61.
85. Lagrotteria D, Holmes S, Smieja M, et al. Prospective, randomized inpatient study of oral metronidazole versus oral metronidazole and rifampin for treatment of primary episode of Clostridium difficile-associated diarrhea. Clin Infect Dis 2006; 43(5):547–52.
86. McFarland LV, Elmer GW, Surawicz CM. Breaking the cycle: treatment strategies for 163 cases of recurrent Clostridium difficile disease. Am J Gastroenterol 2002; 97(7):1769–75.
87. Johnson S, Gerding DN. Fidaxomicin "chaser" regimen following vancomycin for patients with multiple Clostridium difficile recurrences. Clin Infect Dis 2013;56(2): 309–10.
88. van Nood E, Vrieze A, Nieuwdorp M, et al. Duodenal infusion of donor feces for recurrent Clostridium difficile. N Engl J Med 2013;368(5):407–15.
89. Villano SA, Seiberling M, Tatarowicz W, et al. Evaluation of an oral suspension of vp20621, spores of nontoxigenic Clostridium difficile strain m3, in healthy subjects. Antimicrob Agents Chemother 2012;56(10):5224–9.
90. Juang P, Skledar SJ, Zgheib NK, et al. Clinical outcomes of intravenous immune globulin in severe Clostridium difficile-associated diarrhea. Am J Infect Control 2007;35(2):131–7.
91. Wilcox MH. Descriptive study of intravenous immunoglobulin for the treatment of recurrent Clostridium difficile diarrhoea. J Antimicrob Chemother 2004;53(5): 882–4.
92. Kurtz CB, Cannon EP, Brezzani A, et al. Gt160-246, a toxin binding polymer for treatment of Clostridium difficile colitis. Antimicrob Agents Chemother 2001; 45(8):2340–7.

Fecal Microbiota Transplantation for the Management of *Clostridium difficile* Infection

Krishna Rao, MD[a,b], Vincent B. Young, MD, PhD[a,c],*

KEYWORDS

- *Clostridium difficile* • Fecal microbiota transplantation • Microbiome • Colitis
- Recurrent *C difficile* infection • Nonantibiotic treatment

KEY POINTS

- Disruption of the gut microbiome is a prerequisite for *Clostridium difficile* infection (CDI) and can persist after treatment.
- *C difficile* can cause recurrent infection that can be difficult to manage with conventional treatments, which do not restore the microbiome to a healthy state.
- Fecal microbiota transplantation (FMT), which takes stool from a healthy donor and infuses it into the gastrointestinal (GI) tract of the recipient, is highly effective in treating recurrent CDI and is safe in the short term.
- Despite numerous protocols with significant variation in the stool sources, methods for preparation, and routes of instillation, the effectiveness of FMT generally remains high.
- The long-term safety of FMT has not been established, and changes in the microbiome have been associated with several medical conditions.

Conflicts of interest: Authors have no reported conflicts.

Funding: This work was supported by grants from the National Institute of Allergy and Infectious Diseases at the National Institutes of Health (grant number U19-AI090871), the Claude D. Pepper Older Americans Independence Center (grant number AG-024824), and the Michigan Institute for Clinical and Health Research (grant number 2UL1TR000433). The funders had no role in study design, data collection and analysis, decision to publish, or preparation of the article.

[a] Division of Infectious Diseases, Department of Internal Medicine, University of Michigan School of Medicine, 1500 East Medical Center Drive, Ann Arbor, MI 48109, USA; [b] Division of Infectious Diseases, Department of Internal Medicine, Veterans Affairs Ann Arbor Healthcare System, 2215 Fuller Road, Ann Arbor, MI 48105, USA; [c] Department of Microbiology and Immunology, University of Michigan School of Medicine, 1150 West Medical Center Drive, Ann Arbor, MI 48109, USA

* Corresponding author. Division of Infectious Diseases, Department of Internal Medicine, University of Michigan School of Medicine, 1500 East Medical Center Drive, Ann Arbor, MI 48109.

E-mail address: youngvi@umich.edu

Infect Dis Clin N Am 29 (2015) 109–122
http://dx.doi.org/10.1016/j.idc.2014.11.009
0891-5520/15/$ – see front matter

id.theclinics.com

INTRODUCTION: NATURE OF THE PROBLEM

Pathogenesis and Natural History of Clostridium difficile Infection

The human gut microbiota is a diverse ecosystem consisting of thousands of bacterial species.[1] It is thought that one role of this ecosystem is to protect against invasion by pathogens.[2,3] The predominant understanding of the pathogenesis of CDI is that it requires disruption of the gut microbiota as a prerequisite for the onset of symptomatic disease (**Fig. 1**).[4] This disruption usually occurs through exposure to antibiotics, which alter the composition and function of the microbiome to a state susceptible to CDI.[5] After exposure to *C difficile* spores, patients can either become asymptomatically colonized or develop symptomatic infection.[6,7] Colonization follows germination of the *C difficile* spores and vegetative outgrowth. Subsequent expression of the toxins TcdA and TcdB, the main virulence factors of *C difficile*, results in epithelial damage and symptomatic infection. CDI can be self-limited[8,9] but usually requires treatment with antibiotics that have activity against *C difficile*,[10] although the treatments are nonspecific and have activity against other gut bacteria. Features of infection include diarrhea, leukocytosis, fever, or pseudomembranous colitis.[10] Some patients can experience severe disease, including signs and symptoms such as abdominal pain, ileus, or septic shock that results in admission to an intensive care unit (ICU), abdominal surgery such as colectomy, or even death.[11]

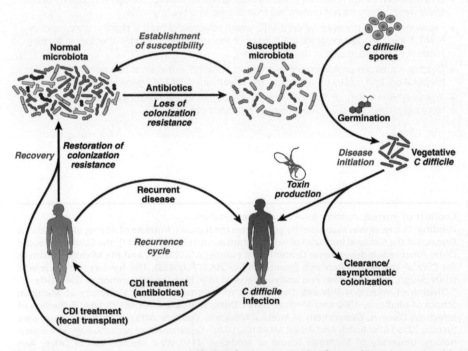

Fig. 1. Pathogenesis of *Clostridium difficile* infection (CDI). This figure shows how a healthy gut microbiota (upper left corner) is altered by antibiotics to a susceptible state in which either asymptomatic colonization or symptomatic CDI can occur. Some patients do not have recovery of the microbiome back to a healthy state and experience recurrent CDI. Fecal microbiota transplantation can help restore the microbiome to a state resistant to CDI. (*Adapted from* Britton RA, Young VB. Role of the intestinal microbiota in resistance to colonization by *Clostridium difficile*. Gastroenterology 2014;146(6):1548; with permission.)

RECURRENT *CLOSTRIDIUM DIFFICILE* INFECTION

After recovery from infection, some patients retain a microbiome susceptible to CDI and can have recurrent disease (see **Fig. 1**),[12] due to either recrudescence of the original infection or reinfection with a new strain.[13] After an initial episode of CDI, 15% to 20% of successfully treated patients suffer a recurrence and up to 45% of those patients can have a second recurrence; however, less than 5% of all patients who have an initial episode of CDI can enter a cycle of recurrent disease with multiple recurrences.[14–16] Conventional therapies for recurrent CDI include extended pulses and/or tapering doses of either metronidazole or (usually) vancomycin.[10,17] Multiple regimens exist and the duration varies from 4 to 10 weeks, followed in some instances by either rifaximin or fidaxomicin as a cap or chaser after initial therapy.[10,18,19] The possible mechanism by which this acts involves agents with a narrower spectrum of antimicrobial activity, allowing the microbiome to recover while still suppressing *C difficile* activity.

Some patients have recurrent CDI recalcitrant to these treatments and relapse soon after antibiotics are stopped. A trial of chronic, low-dose antibiotics to suppress CDI is an option, although there are downsides to this strategy—increased antimicrobial resistance, continued microbiome disruption, and breakthroughs requiring retreatment at higher dosages. Faced with this prospect, other therapeutic options are often discussed in these patients. It is unclear why patients experience recurrent infection, but host factors such as antibody response to toxins,[20] microbial factors such as *C difficile* strain,[21,22] and community factors such as persistent disruption of the gut microbiome[23] all may play a role. Augmentation of the immune response through intravenous infusion of immunoglobulin has variable efficacy.[24] A strain-dependent differential recurrence rate for treatment, either of primary CDI or of a first recurrence, with the antibiotic fidaxomicin has been demonstrated.[12,25] However, it is not clear how this translates into clinical benefit, especially for those with multiple recurrences. Restoration of the gut microbiome is the treatment strategy that has garnered the most attention and has gained acceptance among practitioners for treatment of recurrent CDI.[26]

Role of the Gut Microbiota in Recurrent Clostridium difficile Infection

As noted earlier, disruption of the normal indigenous gut microbiota is a prerequisite for the development of CDI. The potential mechanisms by which the indigenous microbiota normally prevents colonization by pathogens such as *C difficile* are not fully understood. It is likely that multiple mechanisms play a role, including competition for nutritional niches, production of metabolites that are deleterious to *C difficile*, stimulating host immune responses, and modulating the physiology of the pathogen, as summarized in recent reviews.[4,27] Disruption of the indigenous microbiota with antibiotics alters the community structure and function, resulting in the loss of colonization resistance. In patients who are successfully treated for CDI with standard antibiotic therapy, it is assumed that the indigenous microbiota recovers to the point that normal function is restored and colonization resistance returns. In patients who develop recurrent CDI, this functional recovery of the microbiota does not occur. Patients with recurrent CDI have a microbiota characterized by lower-than-normal community diversity (**Fig. 2**).[23] In itself, lowered diversity is not a mechanism that permits continued persistence of *C difficile*; rather, this low diversity is a marker of continued disruption of microbiota community structure and function. This persistence of a structurally and functionally deficient microbiota provides the rationale for use of fecal microbiota transfer to treat recurrent CDI. By providing access to members of the

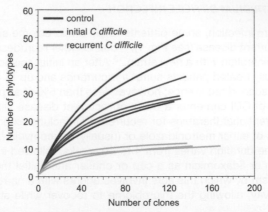

Fig. 2. Diversity of the gut microbiome and recurrent *Clostridium difficile* infection. Rarefaction curve analysis indicates that patients with recurrent infection have lower diversity of their gut microbiome compared with healthy controls or patients with a successfully treated initial infection. (*Adapted from* Chang JY, Antonopoulos DA, Kalra A, et al. Decreased diversity of the fecal microbiome in recurrent *Clostridium difficile*–associated diarrhea. J Infect Dis 2008;197(3):437; with permission.)

microbiota that can carry on specific functions that mediate colonization resistance, FMT can reverse the damage. It has been demonstrated that, after successful FMT for CDI, the patient's stool more closely resembles the composition (and thus the function) of the donated stool (**Fig. 3**).[28]

In addition to the microbial composition of the stool, fecal contents include a wide range of metabolites. The role of these metabolites in symptomatic recovery from recurrent CDI after FMT has not been determined, although data from human studies and animal models describe changes in bile salt composition.[5,29] The nature of these changes in bile salts is uncertain, but they may play a role in immediate symptom relief reported by some patients[30] or be involved in the mechanism by which the microbiome influences subsequent recovery and colonization resistance.

OVERVIEW OF FECAL MICROBIOTA TRANSPLANTATION
Historical Perspective

FMT, which uses healthy stool to restore the microbiome to a state resistant to CDI, has recently reemerged as a safe and effective option for treatment of recurrent CDI. FMT is not new to modern times, as there are reports of its use in ancient China for various purposes.[31] It was first described as a treatment of pseudomembranous colitis in the 1950s[32] and then is not well-described in the literature again until 1983, when Schwann and colleagues[30] published the use of fecal enema to treat a 65-year-old woman with CDI, who had symptomatic resolution within 24 hours. The number of protocols and possible routes of administration increased: Aas and colleagues[33] reported using FMT via nasogastric infusion of stool in 1994; Persky and Brandt[34] performed FMT via colonoscopy in 2000; and in 2010, Silverman and colleagues[35] reported a case series of self-administered FMTs via fecal retention enemas by patients in their own homes. In the past several years, the use of FMT for CDI has become widespread.

Stool Preparation Methods

Preparation and infusion of donor stool for FMT takes myriad forms, as reported in the published protocols.[36–38] Diluents typically include tap water or normal saline, but

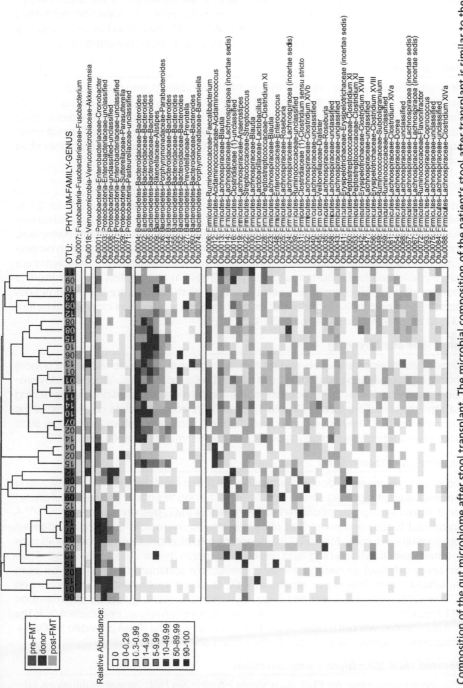

Fig. 3. Composition of the gut microbiome after stool transplant. The microbial composition of the patient's stool after transplant is similar to the donor's stool and is more diverse than before transplant. (*Adapted from* Seekatz AM, Aas J, Gessert CE, et al. Recovery of the gut microbiome following fecal microbiota transplantation. mBio 2014;5(3):e00895; with permission.)

yogurt, milk, and mixtures with psyllium husk have also been used. Some protocols call for gentle agitation of stool with the diluent, while others blend the whole preparation. Often, stool is collected and prepared within hours of administration, but frozen stool preparations collected weeks or months before FMT have also been successfully used.[39] The amount of prepared stool infusate also varies but is generally at least 50 g.

Routes of Instillation

The sites of stool instillation include the stomach, duodenum, and proximal/distal large intestine.[37,38] Infusion into the upper GI tract takes place through a nasogastric or nasojejunal tube or via gastroscopy. Infusion into the lower GI tract takes place using retention enemas, which the patients self-administer in some protocols,[35] or via colonoscopy, which usually infuses the donor stool into the terminal ileum and other sites more distal as the colonoscope is withdrawn.

Recipient Preparation

It is generally recommended that recipients withhold any antibiotic therapy for 24 to 48 hours before FMT, if possible, as presence of antibiotics in the GI tract adversely affects the health of the donated stool and decreases the efficacy of the transplant. A bowel preparation or lavage, often with a solution of polyethylene glycol, can be performed and is especially common in protocols using a colonoscope.[36] Recipients are typically screened for blood-borne pathogens (**Table 1**) to establish whether there is evidence of prior infection, which can be helpful post-FMT if a transmission is suspected. Some protocols call for use of an antimotility agent such as loperamide before FMT, to aid in retention of the transplant.[36]

Donor Type and Screening

Donor eligibility also varies between protocols. In general, it is preferred to use donors who are in generally good health and have normal bowel movements. Although many protocols use donors known to the patients, some use universal standard donors. Screening tests typically used are listed in **Table 1**. In addition, some absolute contraindications to donation for FMT have been proposed (**Table 2**), including high-risk behaviors such as intravenous drug use and conditions such as inflammatory bowel disease (IBD).

Synthetic Stool/Frozen Stool

Use of a single universal donor is attractive, as it can expedite the FMT process and obviates frequent repeated screenings. In lieu of having this donor provide stool on demand, frozen stool preparations have been used for FMT, even in capsule form.[39,40] A clinical trial is also underway that uses a synthetic microbiota suspension, derived from intestinal sources, for FMT.[41] A nonprofit organization, OpenBiome, takes care of donor selection/screening and stool preparation (www.OpenBiome.org). They ship prepared stool for nasogastric or colonoscopic administration that can be used immediately after thawing or stored at −20°C for up to 6 months. The proposed 2014 revision to the US Food and Drug Administration (FDA) guidance statement on FMT requires that the donor be known to the treating physician or recipient.[42] If the draft is accepted without modification, then services such as those provided by Open-Biome may no longer be available in the United States.

Repeated Fecal Microbiota Transplantations

Although success rates for FMT via a single infusion are high, repeated infusions take place in many protocols and can increase the overall efficacy.[37] Most clinicians do not repeat FMT routinely without evaluating the first FMT for clinical success.

Table 1
Screening tests for potentially transmissible infectious pathogens in donors and recipients undergoing fecal microbiota transplantation

Pathogen/Infection	Usual Tests	Recipient, Donor, or Both	Part of Routine or Extended Screening
Hepatitis A/B/C	Serum antibodies; serum PCR	Both	Routine
HIV	Third- or fourth-generation serum ELISA; serum RNA PCR if recent seroconversion possible	Both	Routine
Syphilis	Nontreponemal serum test followed by treponemal confirmatory test if positive (eg, serum RPR followed by TP-PA)	Both	Routine
Enteric bacterial pathogens (*Salmonella* species, *E coli*, *Shigella* species, and others)	Routine stool culture	Donor	Routine
Enteric helminths and protozoa	Stool microscopy for ova and parasites; antigen ELISAs for *Giardia* and *Cryptosporidium* species	Donor	Routine
Clostridium difficile	Stool EIA for bacterial products and/or PCR	Donor	Routine
Epstein-Barr virus	Serum antibodies; PCR	Both	Extended (HSCT and SOT patients)
Cytomegalovirus	Serum antibodies; PCR	Both	Extended (HSCT and SOT patients)
Others (*Helicobacter pylori*, HTLV, and many others)	Various tests	Usually donor only	Extended (research protocols)

This table outlines the typical screening tests performed for potentially transmissible infectious pathogens in donor stool/circulation. The recipient is also screened in some cases to establish prior infection. Some screening is routine and universal, while other screening is reserved for research or protocols using a single common donor.

Abbreviations: EIA, enzyme immunoassay; ELISA, enzyme-linked immunosorbent assay; HIV, human immunodeficiency virus; HSCT, hematopoietic stem cell transplant; HTLV, human T-lymphotropic virus; PCR, polymerase chain reaction; RNA, ribonucleic acid; RPR, rapid plasma reagent; SOT, solid-organ transplant; TP-PA, *Treponema pallidum* particle agglutination.

CLINICAL OUTCOMES FROM FECAL MICROBIOTA TRANSPLANTATION FOR RECURRENT *CLOSTRIDIUM DIFFICILE* INFECTION
Case Series and Case Reports

Two large systematic reviews of FMT for CDI have been published.[37,38] The first, by Gough and colleagues,[37] included published articles, abstracts from conference proceedings, and unpublished data solicited from investigators. This comprehensive search included case data on 317 patients treated via FMT for recurrent CDI, but no controlled trials were found. The routes used for FMT included distal infusion into the GI tract via retention enema (35%) or colonoscopy (42%) and proximal infusion via nasogastric/nasojejunal tube or gastroscope (23%). The investigators did look at some of the variability in protocols and found differences in resolution rates: infusion into the upper GI tract (76%) versus lower GI tract (89%–96%), related donors (93%)

Table 2
Proposed contraindications to donation for fecal microbiota transplantation

Risk Factor/Condition	Absolute or Relative Contraindication
Known HIV or viral hepatitis infection or recent exposure (12 mo)	Absolute
High-risk sexual behaviors (sexual contact with someone infected with HIV/viral hepatitis, men who have sex with men, sex for money)	Absolute
Use of illicit drugs	Relative (can consider if in remission and in distant past)
Recent tattoo or body piercing (12 mo)	Relative
Incarceration or history of incarceration	Relative
Risk factors for Creutzfeldt-Jakob disease	Absolute
Recent travel (6 mo) to regions where endemic diarrheal illness is prevalent	Relative
Past or present irritable bowel syndrome, inflammatory bowel disease, or gastrointestinal malignancy/known polyposis	Absolute
Recent antibiotic use (3–6 mo or more)	Absolute (consider delaying FMT if able and another donor unavailable)
Ingestion of allergen with known recipient allergy (eg, tree nuts)	Relative (delay FMT if recent ingestion and donor abstains)
Others (eg, metabolic syndrome, major gastrointestinal surgery [such as gastric bypass], systemic autoimmune disease, atopic disorders [asthma, eczema, eosinophilic disorders of the gastrointestinal tract])	Relative/unknown

versus unrelated donors (84%), male donors (86%) versus female donors (100%), tap water as a diluent (99%) versus saline (86%), and volume of FMT infusate greater than 500 mL (97%) versus less than 500 mL (80%). Although these findings are interesting, it is not possible to draw any definite conclusions, as that would require controlled trials examining each of the variables.

Regardless of this variability, 92% of patients overall had resolution of their recurrent CDI after one or, from these data, more treatments. After only 1 treatment, 89% had resolution of symptoms. Of the 4% of patients who had relapsed CDI after the first FMT, 87.5% had resolution after one or more repeat FMTs.

A second review by Kassam and colleagues[38] in 2013 was more limited in scope as the investigators included only completed, published studies that were peer reviewed and had a sample size of 10 or more patients. Similar to the review by Gough and colleagues,[37] of the 273 patients included in this review, 89.7% had resolution of CDI with FMT. A subgroup analysis showed that FMT into the lower GI tract had a higher resolution rate (91.4%) than FMT into the upper GI tract (82.3%).

Another systematic review of FMT in general, not just for CDI, reinforced the overall efficacy and benign safety profile of FMT for CDI.[43] Other individual case series and reports not included in these reviews have been published, but they are all similar in finding an excellent resolution rate for CDI treated by FMT.[39,44–48]

Clinical Trials

In 2013, van Nood and colleagues[49] published the first randomized controlled trial on FMT for recurrent CDI via duodenal infusion. Patients were randomized to receive vancomycin for 5 days followed by FMT ($n = 16$), vancomycin alone for 14 days ($n = 13$), or vancomycin for 14 days with bowel lavage (rapid administration of a large volume of polyethylene glycol solution) ($n = 13$). The primary outcome was cure defined as absence of diarrhea or persistent diarrhea from another cause, with 3 consecutive stool tests negative for *C difficile* toxin. The study was stopped early after an interim analysis, as 94% of patients in the FMT group achieved cure (81% were cured after 1 infusion) versus 31% or 23% in the vancomycin alone or vancomycin with bowel lavage groups, respectively. Based on these findings, off-protocol FMT was offered to 18 patients in the other treatment arms, and this achieved an 83% cure rate.

In a pilot trial published by Youngster and colleagues,[50] patients were randomized to receive FMT via either colonoscopy or nasogastric tube from a frozen fecal suspension. A total of only 10 patients in each arm were enrolled, but they did not show a statistically significant difference in efficacy between administration routes. Following this, Youngster and colleagues[40] conducted an open-label feasibility study using frozen fecal capsules for FMT in 20 patients with 3 or more episodes of CDI and failure of vancomycin taper(s) or 2 or more episodes of severe CDI requiring hospitalization. Resolution occurred in 14 (70%) patients after a single treatment, and 4 of the 6 nonresponders had resolution on retreatment for an overall efficacy of 90%. There are several other clinical trials studying FMT for CDI underway that are not yet completed.[41,51–55]

Other Clostridium difficile Infection-Related Indications

The success of FMT in treating recurrent CDI has spurred interest in its role in treating primary CDI or severe CDI. Few data exist for the use of FMT in primary CDI. Lofgren and colleagues[56] constructed a mathematical model of CDI in an ICU and assessed the role of various treatments, including FMT, on primary CDI. The investigators showed that, compared with conventional treatments the model predicted a decreased median incidence of recurrent CDI in patients with primary CDI treated by FMT. In addition to being a mathematical model and not a real-world study, there were several limitations to the model itself that make it difficult to draw general conclusions about FMT for primary CDI.[57] FMT for severe disease also has been little described in the literature. Although several published case reports suggest that it is effective,[58–61] one recent documented death after FMT for severe CDI underscores the need for more research into the safety and efficacy of FMT for this indication.[62]

COMPLICATIONS AND CONCERNS WITH FECAL MICROBIOTA TRANSPLANTATION FOR CLOSTRIDIUM DIFFICILE INFECTION
Short-term Complications

In all the published literature noted earlier, there were no serious adverse effects directly attributable to FMT, but symptoms of an irritable colon (constipation, diarrhea, cramping, bloating) were reported shortly after FMT and were usually transient (<48 hours).[37] In the special population of immunocompromised patients, CDI has demonstrated safety overall; however, patients with IBD may be at increased risk of adverse events. A recent case series focusing on immunocompromised patients reported that 14% of patients with IBD experienced a disease flare after FMT for CDI, some requiring hospitalization.[45] No cases of infectious complications such as septicemia were reported. Other studies have also found an increased risk of IBD flare or other symptoms such as fever and elevated inflammatory markers after FMT, both for CDI and for other indications.[63–65] Deaths involving FMT have been reported: one death occurred from aspiration pneumonia during sedation for colonoscopy for

FMT,[45] although this was not directly related to the procedure. In a more concerning case, one patient with severe CDI failed FMT and died afterward from toxic megacolon and shock, although it is uncertain whether and to what degree FMT or withdrawal of antibiotics with activity against CDI after FMT contributed to the outcome.[62] Although some evidence for safety exists, FMT is largely untested in patients with severe CDI[58–61] and the fatal case of toxic megacolon noted earlier is of concern. One study of a single-agent probiotic in critically ill patients with acute pancreatitis found an increase in mortality,[66] raising the concern for use of probiotics or FMT in patients in the ICU. Further research is needed to determine if FMT for severe CDI has an acceptable safety profile.

Long-term Complications

Although safe in most patients in the short run, the long-term safety profile of FMT has yet to be established. Some of the concern over the safety of FMT stems from an incomplete understanding of the complex interplay between the specific composition of the gut microbiome and the host. The intestinal microbiota has been associated with colon cancer, diabetes, obesity, and atopic disorders such as asthma.[67] Whether FMT can place the recipient at increased risk of developing these conditions and if proper screening and selection of donor stool can mitigate such risk are unknown.

One study evaluated 77 patients in terms of efficacy and safety 3 to 68 months (mean 17 months) after FMT.[68] Although the scope of the primary survey was limited to symptoms and recurrence of CDI, some patients did report the development of new conditions, including autoimmune disease, ovarian cancer, myocardial infarction, and stroke. These concerns underscore the need for more longitudinal studies on patients who have undergone FMT.

Regulatory Environment

FMT has now become accepted and is in widespread use, drawing the attention of the United States Department of Health and Human Services' FDA in 2013, which published guidance suggesting that stool should be regulated as a biologic agent.[69] The FDA feels that an Investigational New Drug application is required for FMT but intends to exercise enforcement discretion in certain use situations, such as treatment of recurrent CDI. The FDA had planned to revise this guidance statement in 2014 but has not yet finalized the policy (as of December 18, 2014).[42]

SUMMARY

Both among physicians and patients, there has been a growing acceptance of FMT as a viable treatment option for recurrent CDI.[26,70] Performing FMT does involve choosing among numerous specific parameters and navigating some logistic hurdles. These include informed consent; donor type, selection, and screening; preparation of the stool for infusion; and route of administration. Despite the numerous options for these parameters, the overall efficacy of FMT remains high. Although in the short term FMT seems to be safe, the long-term safety has not yet been established. Fewer data on the use of FMT for primary CDI or severe CDI exist. The regulatory status of FMT in the United States, especially concerning stool banks, is not solidly defined and remains in flux, but this has not discouraged its widespread use.

REFERENCES

1. Yatsunenko T, Rey FE, Manary MJ, et al. Human gut microbiome viewed across age and geography. Nature 2012;486(7402):222–7.

2. Van der Waaij D, Berghuis-de Vries JM, Lekkerkerk-van der Wees JE. Colonization resistance of the digestive tract in conventional and antibiotic-treated mice. Epidemiol Infect 1971;69(03):405–11.
3. Vollaard E, Clasener H. Colonization resistance. Antimicrob Agents Chemother 1994;38(3):409.
4. Britton RA, Young VB. Role of the intestinal microbiota in resistance to colonization by *Clostridium difficile*. Gastroenterology 2014;146(6):1547–53.
5. Theriot CM, Koenigsknecht MJ, Carlson PE Jr, et al. Antibiotic-induced shifts in the mouse gut microbiome and metabolome increase susceptibility to *Clostridium difficile* infection. Nat Commun 2014;5:3114.
6. Samore MH, DeGirolami PC, Tlucko A, et al. *Clostridium difficile* colonization and diarrhea at a tertiary care hospital. Clin Infect Dis 1994;18(2):181–7.
7. Riggs MM, Sethi AK, Zabarsky TF, et al. Asymptomatic carriers are a potential source for transmission of epidemic and nonepidemic *Clostridium difficile* strains among long-term care facility residents. Clin Infect Dis 2007;45(8):992–8.
8. Bartlett JG. Treatment of antibiotic-associated pseudomembranous colitis. Rev Infect Dis 1984;6(Suppl 1):S235–41.
9. Olson MM, Shanholtzer CJ, Lee JT Jr, et al. Ten years of prospective *Clostridium difficile*-associated disease surveillance and treatment at the Minneapolis VA Medical Center, 1982-1991. Infect Control Hosp Epidemiol 1994;15(6):371–81.
10. Debast SB, Bauer MP, Kuijper EJ. European Society of Clinical Microbiology and Infectious Diseases: update of the treatment guidance document for *Clostridium difficile* infection. Clin Microbiol Infect 2014;20(Suppl 2):1–26.
11. McDonald LC, Coignard B, Dubberke E, et al. Recommendations for surveillance of *Clostridium difficile*-associated disease. Infect Control Hosp Epidemiol 2007; 28(2):140–5.
12. Figueroa I, Johnson S, Sambol SP, et al. Relapse versus reinfection: recurrent *Clostridium difficile* infection following treatment with fidaxomicin or vancomycin. Clin Infect Dis 2012;55(Suppl 2):S104–9.
13. Eyre DW, Babakhani F, Griffiths D, et al. Whole-genome sequencing demonstrates that fidaxomicin is superior to vancomycin for preventing reinfection and relapse of infection with *Clostridium difficile*. J Infect Dis 2014;209(9): 1446–51.
14. Bakken JS. Fecal bacteriotherapy for recurrent *Clostridium difficile* infection. Anaerobe 2009;15(6):285–9.
15. Huebner ES, Surawicz CM. Treatment of recurrent *Clostridium difficile* diarrhea. Gastroenterol Hepatol 2006;2(3):203–8.
16. Borody TJ, Warren EF, Leis SM, et al. Bacteriotherapy using fecal flora: toying with human motions. J Clin Gastroenterol 2004;38(6):475–83.
17. McFarland LV, Elmer GW, Surawicz CM. Breaking the cycle: treatment strategies for 163 cases of recurrent *Clostridium difficile* disease. Am J Gastroenterol 2002; 97(7):1769–75.
18. Garey KW, Ghantoji SS, Shah DN, et al. A randomized, double-blind, placebo-controlled pilot study to assess the ability of rifaximin to prevent recurrent diarrhoea in patients with *Clostridium difficile* infection. J Antimicrob Chemother 2011;66(12):2850–5.
19. Johnson S, Gerding DN. Fidaxomicin 'chaser' regimen following vancomycin for patients with multiple *C. difficile* recurrences. Clin Infect Dis 2012;56(2):309–10.
20. Kyne L, Warny M, Qamar A, et al. Association between antibody response to toxin A and protection against recurrent *Clostridium difficile* diarrhoea. Lancet 2001; 357(9251):189–93.

21. Crook DW, Walker AS, Kean Y, et al. Fidaxomicin versus vancomycin for *Clostridium difficile* infection: meta-analysis of pivotal randomized controlled trials. Clin Infect Dis 2012;55(Suppl 2):S93–103.
22. Abou Chakra CN, Pepin J, Sirard S, et al. Risk factors for recurrence, complications and mortality in *Clostridium difficile* infection: a systematic review. PLoS One 2014;9(6):e98400.
23. Chang JY, Antonopoulos DA, Kalra A, et al. Decreased diversity of the fecal microbiome in recurrent *Clostridium difficile*–associated diarrhea. J Infect Dis 2008; 197(3):435–8.
24. O'Horo J, Safdar N. The role of immunoglobulin for the treatment of *Clostridium difficile* infection: a systematic review. Int J Infect Dis 2009;13(6):663–7.
25. Cornely OA, Miller MA, Louie TJ, et al. Treatment of first recurrence of *Clostridium difficile* infection: fidaxomicin versus vancomycin. Clin Infect Dis 2012;55(Suppl 2):S154–61.
26. Bakken JS, Polgreen PM, Beekmann SE, et al. Treatment approaches including fecal microbiota transplantation for recurrent *Clostridium difficile* infection (RCDI) among infectious disease physicians. Anaerobe 2013;24:20–4.
27. Britton RA, Young VB. Interaction between the intestinal microbiota and host in *Clostridium difficile* colonization resistance. Trends Microbiol 2012;20(7): 313–9.
28. Seekatz AM, Aas J, Gessert CE, et al. Recovery of the gut microbiome following fecal microbiota transplantation. MBio 2014;5(3):e00893–914.
29. Weingarden AR, Chen C, Bobr A, et al. Microbiota transplantation restores normal fecal bile acid composition in recurrent *Clostridium difficile* infection. Am J Physiol Gastrointest Liver Physiol 2014;306(4):G310–9.
30. Schwan A, Sjolin S, Trottestam U, et al. Relapsing *Clostridium difficile* enterocolitis cured by rectal infusion of homologous faeces. Lancet 1983;322(8354):845.
31. Zhang F, Luo W, Shi Y, et al. Should we standardize the 1,700-year-old fecal microbiota transplantation? Am J Gastroenterol 2012;107(11):1755.
32. Eiseman B, Silen W, Bascom GS, et al. Fecal enema as an adjunct in the treatment of pseudomembranous enterocolitis. Surgery 1958;44(5):854–9.
33. Aas J, Gessert CE, Bakken JS. Recurrent *Clostridium difficile* colitis: case series involving 18 patients treated with donor stool administered via a nasogastric tube. Clin Infect Dis 2003;36(5):580–5.
34. Persky SE, Brandt LJ. Treatment of recurrent *Clostridium difficile*–associated diarrhea by administration of donated stool directly through a colonoscope. Am J Gastroenterol 2000;95(11):3283–5.
35. Silverman MS, Davis I, Pillai DR. Success of self-administered home fecal transplantation for chronic *Clostridium difficile* infection. Clin Gastroenterol Hepatol 2010;8(5):471–3.
36. Bakken JS, Borody T, Brandt LJ, et al. Treating *Clostridium difficile* infection with fecal microbiota transplantation. Clin Gastroenterol Hepatol 2011;9(12):1044–9.
37. Gough E, Shaikh H, Manges AR. Systematic review of intestinal microbiota transplantation (fecal bacteriotherapy) for recurrent *Clostridium difficile* infection. Clin Infect Dis 2011;53(10):994–1002.
38. Kassam Z, Lee CH, Yuan Y, et al. Fecal microbiota transplantation for *Clostridium difficile* infection: systematic review and meta-analysis. Am J Gastroenterol 2013; 108(4):500–8.
39. Hamilton MJ, Weingarden AR, Sadowsky MJ, et al. Standardized frozen preparation for transplantation of fecal microbiota for recurrent *Clostridium difficile* infection. Am J Gastroenterol 2012;107(5):761–7.

40. Youngster I, Russell GH, Pindar C, et al. Oral, capsulized, frozen fecal microbiota transplantation for relapsing *Clostridium difficile* infection. JAMA 2014;312(17): 1772–8. http://dx.doi.org/10.1001/jama.2014.13875.

41. Rebiotix Inc. Microbiota restoration therapy for recurrent *Clostridium difficile*-associated diarrhea (PUNCH CD). ClinicalTrials.gov. [Internet]. Bethesda (MD): National Library of Medicine (US); 2000. Available at: http://clinicaltrials.gov/ct2/show/NCT01925417. Accessed July 1, 2014. NLM Identifier: NCT01925417.

42. Draft guidance for industry: enforcement policy regarding investigational new drug requirements for use of fecal microbiota for transplantation to treat *Clostridium difficile* infection not responsive to standard therapies. U.S. Department of Health and Human Services, Food and Drug Administration. Available at: http://www.fda.gov/biologicsbloodvaccines/guidancecomplianceregulatoryinformation/guidances/vaccines/ucm387023.htm. Accessed July 1, 2014.

43. Sha S, Liang J, Chen M, et al. Systematic review: faecal microbiota transplantation therapy for digestive and nondigestive disorders in adults and children. Aliment Pharmacol Ther 2014;39(10):1003–32.

44. Kassam Z, Hundal R, Marshall JK, et al. Fecal transplant via retention enema for refractory or recurrent *Clostridium difficile* infection. Arch Intern Med 2012;172(2):191–3.

45. Kelly CR, Ihunnah C, Fischer M, et al. Fecal microbiota transplant for treatment of *Clostridium difficile* infection in immunocompromised patients. Am J Gastroenterol 2014;109(7):1065–71.

46. Dutta SK, Girotra M, Garg S, et al. Efficacy of combined jejunal and colonic fecal microbiota transplantation for recurrent *Clostridium difficile* infection. Clin Gastroenterol Hepatol 2014;12(9):1572–6.

47. Friedman-Moraco RJ, Mehta AK, Lyon GM, et al. Fecal microbiota transplantation for refractory *Clostridium difficile* colitis in solid organ transplant recipients. Am J Transplant 2014;14(2):477–80.

48. Emanuelsson F, Claesson BE, Ljungström L, et al. Faecal microbiota transplantation and bacteriotherapy for recurrent *Clostridium difficile* infection: a retrospective evaluation of 31 patients. Scand J Infect Dis 2014;46(2):89–97.

49. van Nood E, Vrieze A, Nieuwdorp M, et al. Duodenal Infusion of Donor Feces for Recurrent Clostridium difficile. N Engl J Med 2013;368(5):407–15.

50. Youngster I, Sauk J, Pindar C, et al. Fecal microbiota transplant for relapsing *Clostridium difficile* infection using a frozen inoculum from unrelated donors: a randomized, open-label, controlled pilot study. Clin Infect Dis 2014;58(11):1515–22.

51. University Health Network Toronto. Oral vancomycin followed by fecal transplant versus tapering oral vancomycin. ClinicalTrials.gov. [Internet]. Bethesda (MD): National Library of Medicine (US); 2000. Available at: http://clinicaltrials.gov/ct2/show/NCT01226992. Accessed July 1, 2014. NLM Identifier: NCT01226992.

52. Tel-Aviv Sourasky Medical Center. Transplantation of fecal microbiota for *Clostridium difficile* infection. ClinicalTrials.gov. [Internet]. Bethesda (MD): National Library of Medicine (US); 2000. Available at: http://clinicaltrials.gov/ct2/show/NCT01958463. Accessed July 1, 2014. NLM Identifier: NCT01958463.

53. Hadassah Medical Organization. Efficacy and safety of fecal microbiota transplantation for severe *Clostridium difficile* associated colitis. ClinicalTrials.gov. [Internet]. Bethesda (MD): National Library of Medicine (US); 2000. Available at: http://clinicaltrials.gov/ct2/show/NCT01959048. Accessed July 1, 2014. NLM Identifier: NCT01959048.

54. University Hospital Tuebingen. Fecal microbiota transplantation in recurrent or refractory *Clostridium difficile* colitis (TOCSIN). ClinicalTrials.gov. [Internet]. Bethesda (MD): National Library of Medicine (US); 2000. Available at: http://

clinicaltrials.gov/ct2/show/NCT01942447. Accessed July 1, 2014. NLM Identifier: NCT01942447.

55. Duke University. Stool transplants to treat refractory *Clostridium difficile* colitis. ClinicalTrials.gov. [Internet]. Bethesda (MD): National Library of Medicine (US); 2000. Available at: http://clinicaltrials.gov/ct2/show/NCT02127398. Accessed July 1, 2014. NLM Identifier: NCT02127398.

56. Lofgren ET, Moehring RW, Anderson DJ, et al. A mathematical model to evaluate the routine use of fecal microbiota transplantation to prevent incident and recurrent *Clostridium difficile* infection. Infect Control Hosp Epidemiol 2013;35(1): 18–27.

57. Rao K, Young VB, Aronoff DM. Commentary: fecal microbiota therapy: ready for prime time? Infect Control Hosp Epidemiol 2014;35(1):28–30.

58. Neemann K, Eichele DD, Smith PW, et al. Fecal microbiota transplantation for fulminant *Clostridium difficile* infection in an allogeneic stem cell transplant patient. Transpl Infect Dis 2012;14(6):E161–5.

59. Trubiano JA, Gardiner B, Kwong JC, et al. Faecal microbiota transplantation for severe *Clostridium difficile* infection in the intensive care unit. Eur J Gastroenterol Hepatol 2013;25(2):255–7.

60. Gallegos-Orozco J, Paskvan-Gawryletz C, Gurudu S, et al. Successful colonoscopic fecal transplant for severe acute *Clostridium difficile* pseudomembranous colitis. Rev Gastroenterol Mex 2011;77(1):40–2.

61. You DM, Franzos MA, Holman RP. Successful treatment of fulminant *Clostridium difficile* infection with fecal bacteriotherapy. Ann Intern Med 2008;148(8):632–3.

62. Solari PR, Fairchild PG, Noa LJ, et al. Tempered enthusiasm for fecal transplant. Clin Infect Dis 2014;59(2):319.

63. De Leon LM, Watson JB, Kelly CR. Transient flare of ulcerative colitis after fecal microbiota transplantation for recurrent *Clostridium difficile* infection. Clin Gastroenterol Hepatol 2013;11(8):1036–8.

64. Angelberger S, Reinisch W, Makristathis A, et al. Temporal bacterial community dynamics vary among ulcerative colitis patients after fecal microbiota transplantation. Am J Gastroenterol 2013;108(10):1620–30.

65. Kump PK, Gröchenig HP, Lackner S, et al. Alteration of intestinal dysbiosis by fecal microbiota transplantation does not induce remission in patients with chronic active ulcerative colitis. Inflamm Bowel Dis 2013;19(10):2155–65.

66. Besselink MG, van Santvoort HC, Buskens E, et al. Probiotic prophylaxis in predicted severe acute pancreatitis: a randomised, double-blind, placebo-controlled trial. Lancet 2008;371(9613):651–9.

67. Sekirov I, Russell SL, Antunes LC, et al. Gut microbiota in health and disease. Physiol Rev 2010;90(3):859–904.

68. Brandt LJ, Aroniadis OC, Mellow M, et al. Long-term follow-up of colonoscopic fecal microbiota transplant for recurrent *Clostridium difficile* infection. Am J Gastroenterol 2012;107(7):1079–87.

69. Guidance for industry: enforcement policy regarding investigational new drug requirements for use of fecal microbiota for transplantation to treat *Clostridium difficile* infection not responsive to standard therapies. U.S. Department of Health and Human Services, Food and Drug Administration. Available at: http://www.fda.gov/biologicsbloodvaccines/guidancecomplianceregulatoryinformation/guidances/vaccines/ucm361379.htm. Accessed July 1, 2014.

70. Zipursky JS, Sidorsky TI, Freedman CA, et al. Patient attitudes toward the use of fecal microbiota transplantation in the treatment of recurrent *Clostridium difficile* infection. Clin Infect Dis 2012;55(12):1652–8.

The Morbidity, Mortality, and Costs Associated with *Clostridium difficile* Infection

Jennie H. Kwon, DO[a],*, Margaret A. Olsen, PhD, MPH[b],
Erik R. Dubberke, MD, MSPH[c]

KEYWORDS

- *Clostridium difficile* • Morbidity • Mortality • Costs

KEY POINTS

- The morbidity associated with *Clostridium difficile* infection (CDI) includes colectomies, outbreaks, recurrent CDI, discharge to long-term care facilities, and readmissions to the hospital.
- The CDI-attributable mortality before 2000 was 1.5% or less. Since 2000, the CDI-attributable mortality ranges from 4.5% to 5.7% in endemic periods.
- CDI-attributable mortality during epidemic periods ranges from 6.9% to 16.7%.
- The CDI-attributable acute care hospital costs are $3427 to $9960 per episode as estimated by studies adjusting for cost by propensity score matching.

INTRODUCTION

Once thought to be an inconvenient complication of antimicrobials, *Clostridium difficile* is now the most common pathogen to cause health care–associated infections (HAIs) in the United States.[1-9] *C difficile* infection (CDI) is currently well recognized as a cause of significant patient morbidity and mortality and a major burden to the health care system. Initially, the changes in CDI incidence were noted in dramatic outbreaks of CDI. However, increases in the morbidity, mortality, and costs associated with CDI have been noted in endemic settings. In this review, the authors discuss the morbidity, mortality, and burden of CDI in North America to patients and the health care system.

Disclosure statement: No disclosures (J.H. Kwon); Research: Sanofi-Pasteur, Cubist; Consultant: Sanofi-Pasteur, Merck, Pfizer (M.A. Olsen); Research: Sanofi-Pasteur, Merck, Cubist, Microdermis, Rebiotix; Consultant: Sanofi-Pasteur, Merck, Cubist, Rebiotix (E.R. Dubberke).
[a] Division of Infectious Diseases, Washington University School of Medicine, 660 South Euclid Avenue, Box 8051, St Louis, MO 63110, USA; [b] Divisions of Infectious Diseases and Public Health Sciences, Washington University School of Medicine, 660 South Euclid Avenue, Box 8051, St Louis, MO 63110, USA; [c] Division of Infectious Diseases, Section of Transplant Infectious Diseases, Washington University School of Medicine, 660 South Euclid Avenue, Box 8051, St Louis, MO 63110, USA
* Corresponding author.
E-mail address: jkwon@dom.wustl.edu

Infect Dis Clin N Am 29 (2015) 123–134
http://dx.doi.org/10.1016/j.idc.2014.11.003
0891-5520/15/$ – see front matter © 2015 Elsevier Inc. All rights reserved.

id.theclinics.com

MORBIDITY

The burden of CDI in North America has been increasing, and recent data suggest that *C difficile* has replaced *Staphylococcus aureus* as the most common cause of HAIs.[4,9] Miller and colleagues[10] compared the rates of hospital-onset, health care–associated CDI with the rates of HAIs caused by methicillin-resistant *Staphylococcus aureus* (MRSA) and other HAIs at 39 hospitals. Notably, the rates of CDI exceeded MRSA-HAI rates by 25% from 2008 to 2009.[4] In further support of this trend, a recent prevalence survey by Magill and colleagues[9] of 183 US hospitals found that *C difficile* (12.1%) was the most common single organism causing HAIs, with *Staphylococcus aureus* (10.7%) the second most common pathogen.

The authors commonly hear from their patients that CDI is one of the worst, if not *the* worst, conditions that they have experienced. Despite these anecdotal reports, there are limited data that detail the impact of CDI on the patients' health trajectory, functional status, and quality of life. Adverse effects of CDI include colectomies, recurrent CDI, readmissions to the hospital, and discharge to long-term care facilities (LCTF). An understanding of these complications offers a more nuanced appreciation of the experiences of the patients with CDI.

It is difficult to quantify the proportion of patients with severe CDI because a variety of definitions have been used to define severity. Severity has been defined based on laboratory and/or physical examination findings, intensive care unit (ICU) stay, colectomy, and/or mortality. Given this variability, the authors used colectomy rates as an objective indicator of severity across studies (**Table 1**). Before the early 2000s, reported colectomy rates ranged from 0.48% to 1.3%.[1,11] Beginning in 2000, several groups from North America and Europe reported dramatic increases in CDI severity and need for colectomy during CDI epidemics.[1,5,11–14] Dallal and colleagues[1] described an increase in CDI incidence from a baseline of 0.68% of all admissions between 1989 and 1999 to 1.2% of all admissions in 2000.[1] The proportion of patients who underwent a colectomy or died increased from 1.6% to 3.2%.[1] A report from Muto and colleagues[12] from the same institution indicates the incidence of colectomy continued to increase, with 6.2% of patients with CDI from 2000 to 2001 requiring an emergency colectomy.[1,12,15]

A similar experience was reported at the Centre Hospitalier Universitaire de Sherbrooke in Quebec, Canada.[11] From 2003 to 2006, 16.4% of 843 patients developed severe CDI and 1.8% required colectomies, up from 1.3% between 1991 and 2002. By 2004, increases in CDI incidence and severity were noted at multiple hospitals in Quebec.[5] The combined CDI incidence at the 12 hospitals was 22.5 per 1000 admissions, approximately 4 times greater than described in a 1997 Canadian Nosocomial Infection Surveillance Program (CNISP) survey.[5] In the 2004 Quebec outbreak, 1.9% of patients underwent a colectomy and 6.5% of patients required ICU care.[5]

McDonald and colleagues[16] analyzed *C difficile* isolates from 2000 to 2003 in US hospitals where outbreaks occurred and found that the North American pulsed field gel electrophoresis (NAP) 1, restriction enzyme analysis type B1, polymerase chain reaction ribotype 027 (NAP1/B1/027) strain, a previously uncommon strain, accounted for more than 50% of the isolates. This strain was the cause of 82% of CDI cases at the 12 hospitals in Quebec.[5,16] In retrospect, the study by Dallal and colleagues[1] was likely the first report of an epidemic caused by the NAP1/B1/027 strain of CDI.

Fortunately, colectomy rates after 2000 do not seem to have remained persistently elevated in endemic settings (see **Table 1**).[17–21] A multicenter study of tertiary care academic centers from 2000 to 2006 reported that 0.87% of patients with CDI underwent colectomy, with no increases in the colectomy rate during the 7-year time period.[17]

Table 1
Colectomy rates in hospitalized patients with CDI

Reference	Study Time Period	Study Population	Number of Patients with CDI (CDI Incidence)	% Colectomy
Endemic Periods				
Dallal et al[1]	1989–2000	Single institution	2334 (N/A) total from 1989–2000	1999: 0.48%
Pepin et al[11]	1991–2006	1991–2002: single institution	1616 (N/A)	1991–2002: 1.3%
Kasper et al[17]	2000–2006	Multi-institution (n = 5)	8033 (N/A)	0.87%
Gash et al[18]	2006–2007	Single institution	1398 (N/A)	1.3%
Rodriguez et al[19]	2009	Single institution	362 (N/A)	1.0%
Halabi et al[20]	2001–2010	Nationwide Inpatient Sample	2,773,521 (N/A)	0.7%
See et al[21]	2009–2011	Emerging Infections Program	2057 (N/A)	0.3%
Epidemic Periods				
Dallal et al[1]	1989–2000	Single institution	2334 (2000: 1.2%)	2000: 2.6%
Pepin et al[11]	1991–2006	Single institution 2003–2006: NAP1/B1/027: 67%	1616 (N/A)	2003–2006: 1.8%
Muto et al[12]	2000–2001	Single institution REA type 2: 19.5%, REA type 4: 31.5%	419 (0.27%–0.68%)	6.2%
Loo et al[5]	2004	Multi-institution (n = 12) Health care-associated CDI Binary toxin and partial deletion of *tcdC* gene	1703 (2.25%)	1.9%
Dudukgian et al[13,a]	1999–2006	Single institution	398 (N/A)	3.5%
Al-Abed et al[14]	2007–2009	Single institution	528 (N/A)	3.7%

Abbreviations: N/A, not available; NAP, North American pulsed field gel electrophoresis; REA, restriction enzyme analysis.
[a] Although CDI incidence was not provided, Dudukgian and colleagues[13] noted an increase in the proportion of severe cases compared with endemic periods.

This finding is supported by an analysis of the Nationwide Inpatient Sample from 2001 to 2010.[20] Although the colectomy rate initially increased, it leveled off to between 0.85% and 0.89% from 2008 to 2010, with overall 0.7% of people with CDI undergoing colectomy in the 10-year study time period.[20] Although colectomy for CDI can be acutely lifesaving, data indicate that long-term outcomes are poor. Dallas and colleagues[22] followed 61 patients after a colectomy for CDI: 42% of patients died in the hospital, and mortality was 69% at 1 year and 91% at 7 years.[22] The life span of these patients was on average 4 years shorter than expected.[22]

CDI recurrence is another source of morbidity for patients. After an initial diagnosis of CDI, 10% to 30% develop at least one recurrent episode.[23] After a first recurrence, the risk for another recurrence is greater than 40%; after a second recurrence, the risk for a third recurrence is greater than 50%.[24,25] Based on these proportions, approximately 12% of patients with CDI have at least 2 recurrences, and 6% have more than 2 recurrences.[26–28] The Centers for Disease Control and Prevention's Emerging Infections Programs estimated there were 483,120 initial episodes of CDI in the United States in 2011.[29] Considering the frequency of recurrent CDI, there may have been 48,312 to 144,936 people with at least one episode of recurrent CDI in 2011. Conservatively speaking, this suggests there were between 77,299 and 231,898 episodes of recurrent CDI, for 560,419 to 715,018 total cases of CDI in the United States in 2011.

Patients with CDI are more likely to be readmitted to the hospital compared with patients without CDI. In a 2009 Healthcare Cost and Utilization Project (HCUP) statistical brief, 29.1% of patients with CDI were readmitted within 30 days, and 44.8% were readmitted within 90 days.[30] Dubberke and colleagues[3] noted a 52% crude readmission rate and 19% attributable readmission rate within 180 days in patients with CDI versus those without CDI. Because not all readmissions were directly related to a recurrence of CDI in this study, it suggests that CDI contributes to ongoing patient morbidity and an increased risk of hospitalization that extends beyond the acute CDI episode.

Patients with CDI also have an increased likelihood of discharge to LTCFs, providing further evidence that CDI contributes to poor functional status and debilitation.[3] In the HCUP statistical brief, 42% of patients with CDI were discharged to LTCFs, and readmission rates for these patients were higher than the overall patient readmission rate from LTCFs.[30] A multicenter study of mechanically ventilated patients found that patients with CDI were significantly more likely to be discharged to an LCTF than those without CDI (42.4% vs 31.9%).[31] Similarly, in a study of attributable outcomes of CDI in nonsurgical patients, patients with CDI were 1.6 times more likely to be discharged to an LTCF instead of home.[3]

As population-based surveillance for CDI improves, community-associated CDI (CA-CDI) is increasingly being recognized. Patients diagnosed with CA-CDI tend to be younger and healthier than patients with health care–associated CDI (HA-CDI).[32] In a large population-based study of 984 patients with CA-CDI, the median age was 51 years and the median Charlson comorbidity index was 0.[33] Despite the apparent advantage of younger age and healthier status compared with persons with HA-CDI, 25.5% of the patients with CA-CDI required hospitalization.[33] The finding that one-quarter of these relatively young and healthy persons required hospitalization sheds further light on the morbidity of CDI.[33]

MORTALITY

Concomitant with the increase in morbidity related to CDI, there has been an increase in mortality. Before 2000, CDI-attributable mortality seemed to be low (**Table 2**). In 1998, Kyne and colleagues[34] reported no difference in 3-month or

Table 2
Attributable mortality rates in hospitalized patients with CDI

Reference	Study Time Period	Study Population	CDI Category	Number of Patients with CDI (CDI Incidence)	All-Cause Mortality Rate	Attributable Mortality
Endemic Periods						
Miller et al[4]	1997	Multi-institution (n = 19)	HA-CDI	269 (N/A)	15.2% in-hospital	1.5% in-hospital
Dallal et al[1]	1989–2000	Single institution	All in-hospital CDI	2334 (N/A) total from 1989–2000	13.5% in-hospital (1989–2000)	1999: 0.48% in-hospital
Kyne et al[34]	1998	Single institution	HO-CDI	47 (N/A)	N/A	Not associated with excess 90-d or 1-y mortality after adjustments
Dubberke et al[3]	2003	Single institution Nonsurgical patients	All in-hospital CDI	390 (N/A)	38% at 180 d	5.7% at 180 d
Gravel et al[6]	2004–2005	Multi-institution (n = 29) CNISP	HA-CDI	1430 (0.46%)	16.3% at 30 d	5.7% at 30 d
Tabak et al[2]	2007–2008	CareFusion clinical research database	HO-CDI	282 (0.4%)	11.8% in-hospital	4.5% in-hospital
Epidemic Periods						
Dallal et al[1]	1989–2000	Single institution	All in-hospital CDI	343 (2000: 1.2%)		2000: 2.0% in-hospital
Pepin et al[35]	2003–2004	Single institution Epidemic: no strain typing	HO-CDI	161 (0.89%)	23.0% at 30 d 37.3% at 1 y	16.7% at 1 y
Loo et al[5]	2004	Multi-institution (n = 12) Epidemic: binary toxin and partial deletion of *tcdC* gene	HA-CDI	1703 (2.25%)	17.5% at 30 d	6.9% at 30 d

Abbreviations: HO-CDI, health care–onset CDI; N/A, not available.

1-year mortality in patients with CDI compared with uninfected patients with multivariable analysis.[34] In separate studies, Miller and Dallal reported 1.5% and 0.48% in-hospital mortality rates, respectively, suggesting that attributable mortality to CDI was low.[1,4] However, in 2000, Dallal[1] noted that concurrent with the dramatic increases in CDI incidence and severity, the mortality rate increased to 2.0%.[1,3] Likewise, Pepin,[35] in Quebec, found that during their outbreak, the CDI-attributable mortality was 16.7% at 1 year. Even in the short-term in Quebec, Loo and colleagues[5] found a 6.9% CDI-attributable 30-day mortality rate.[5,35]

In contrast to colectomies, CDI-attributable mortality has remained elevated in endemic settings after 2000 compared with before 2000. Dubberke and colleagues'[3] study was the first to identify a statistically significant increase in mortality attributable to CDI (5.7% at 180 days) in an endemic setting. Of note, the increase in mortality was not detected until 45 days after CDI, indicating CDI continues to contribute to patient morbidity and overall decline even after the acute CDI episode.[3] The Canadian CNISP CDI survey was repeated from November 2004 through April 2005, this time with 29 hospitals.[6] A 30-day attributable mortality of 5.7% was identified, an almost 4-fold increase in comparison with the 1997 CNISP survey.[6] More recently, Tabak and colleagues[2] reported a 4.5% CDI-attributable mortality rate from 2007 to 2008 from 6 hospitals in Pennsylvania.

Supporting the impression that CDI continues to contribute to mortality in endemic settings, Hall and colleagues[36] reported that CDI mortality based on death certificate data increased 5-fold from 10/1 million person-years in 2000 to 48/1 million person-years in 2007, with an estimated 14,000 deaths caused by CDI in 2007.[36] In addition, data from the 2011 National Vital Statistics Reports indicate that the age-adjusted death rate caused by CDI (ie, CDI listed as the primary cause of death) was 9.1% higher than in 2010, with CDI ranking as the 17th leading cause of death in the United States in 2011 for the population aged 65 years and older.[37] Zilberberg and colleagues[38] detected a 23% annual increase in CDI hospitalizations from 2000 to 2005 using the Nationwide Inpatient Sample. They also found that the estimated age-adjusted case-fatality rate for CDI hospitalizations almost doubled from 1.2% in 2000 to 2.2% in 2004, indicating the rate of increase in CDI-related deaths exceeded the increase in CDI incidence.[38]

Despite the increases in CDI severity and mortality associated with the emergence of the NAP1/B1/027 strain, data regarding the clinical significance of C difficile strain types and relation to mortality have been conflicting. Walk and colleagues[39] typed isolates from 743 CDI cases from 2010 to 2012 and observed 91 distinct ribotypes, of which 14% were strain 027. After adjusting for microbiologic, epidemiologic, and laboratory covariates, ribotype was not a significant predictor of severe CDI.[39] Other smaller studies have also reported a lack of association between toxin type and mortality.

Conversely, in the CNISP surveillance from 2004 to 2005, 311 (31%) patients were infected with the NAP1/B1/027 strain.[40] Of these 311 patients, 12.5% experienced a severe outcome, compared with 5.9% of the 687 patients infected with other strains.[40] Severe outcomes were defined as ICU admission for CDI, colectomy caused by CDI, or CDI-attributable death.[40]

In further support of the importance between strain type and clinical outcomes, Walker[41] typed 1893 C difficile isolates cultured from toxin enzyme immunoassay–positive stool specimens collected from 2006 to 2011 in Oxfordshire, United Kingdom. Patients infected with clade 5 strains (predominantly ribotype 078, 63 patients, 25% mortality) and clade 2 strains (predominantly ribotype 027, 560 patients, 20% mortality) were significantly more likely to die within 14 days of CDI diagnosis compared with clade 1 strains (1168 patients, 12% mortality) when controlling for other predictors of mortality. This study provides the best evidence to date that strain type is associated with mortality risk. As the largest studies have found associations between strain type and mortality, it is possible the studies that did not identify this association may have not been adequately powered. Other potential explanations include differences in the patient populations studied, timing of diagnosis, differences in circulating strain types, and treatment administered.

COSTS

In addition to CDI-related morbidity and mortality, CDI has a profound economic impact on the health care system. **Table 3** summarizes studies reporting CDI-attributable costs in hospitalized patients, adjusted for inflation to 2012 US dollars (USD). The authors focus their discussion of the cost on the United States because predictors of cost are influenced by the health care system design, and most available studies are from the United States. In these studies, the reported CDI-attributable costs range from $3427 to $33,055.[2,7,8,34,42–45] Reasons for this wide range of cost estimates are likely multifactorial, reflecting the different statistical methods used to calculate attributable costs, number of covariates adjusted for, and the population sampled.

A closer look at the methodology for cost estimation indicates that the use of propensity score matching as well as controlling for a greater number of covariates leads to more conservative estimates of CDI-attributable costs. Patients with CDI often have more comorbidities and a higher severity of underlying illness than patients who do not have CDI. Thus, adjusting for more covariates improves the accuracy of CDI-attributable cost estimates by controlling for more predictors of hospital cost. Propensity score matching involves creating a logistic regression model to predict risk of CDI, followed by matching of cases to uninfected patients based on the likelihood to develop CDI. Propensity score matching may result in more conservative cost estimates because the sickest (and most costly) patients with CDI are more likely to drop out of analysis because they could not be matched to an uninfected patient and, therefore, are not included in the calculation of attributable costs.

Lipp and colleagues[44] used the New York State Department of Health's hospital billing database to determine the hospital costs associated with HA-CDI. Using linear regression and adjusting for a small number of covariates, the estimated cost of CDI was $33,055.[44] Similarly, Pakyz and colleagues[45] analyzed administrative claims data from 45 institutions using linear regression, adjusting for the same type of covariates as Lipp and colleagues, and estimated $32,105 CDI-attributable costs per hospital discharge. Although these two studies produced very similar cost estimates, the use of linear regression and control for few covariates likely resulted in an overestimation of CDI-attributable costs.[44,45]

The range of CDI-attributable costs of the acute care of CDI in studies using propensity score matching is $3427 to $9960.[2,7,8] In the first of the studies to use propensity score matching, Dubberke and colleagues[7] adjusted for greater than 50 variables, estimating $3427 in excess costs caused by CDI per case. Tabak and colleagues[2] adjusted for greater than 30 variables and estimated $6972 attributable costs per case of HO-CDI. Stewart and Hollenbeak[8] used propensity score matching but adjusted for only 7 variables, estimating $9960 per case.[8] This higher estimate may be caused by the smaller number of variables adjusted.

Table 3
Hospital costs and hospital length of stay attributable to CDI

Reference	CDI Category	Year Cost Reported	Study Population	Attributable LOS (d)	Method of Cost Adjustments	Number of Variables Adjusted	Cost Estimate/ Case in USD[a]	Cost Estimate/ Case in 2012 USD[b]
Dubberke et al[7]	All in-hospital CDI	2003	Single institution Nonsurgical patients	2.8	Propensity score match	>50	2454	3427
Song et al[43]	All in-hospital CDI	2005	Single institution	5.5	Direct variable costs, simple matching	6	6326	16,242 (8121)[c]
O'Brien et al[42]	All in-hospital CDI	2005	Massachusetts hospital discharge data	3.9[d]	1° Diagnosis: total costs 2° Diagnosis: adjusted to proportion of stay	N/A	12,703[d]	16,307
Stewart & Hollenbeak[8]	All in-hospital CDI	2007	Nationwide Inpatient Sample	5.0	Propensity score match	7	8426	9960
Lipp et al[44]	HA-CDI	2008	New York Statewide Planning and Research Cooperative System database	12.0	Generalized linear model	6	29,000	33,055
Kyne et al[34]	HO-CDI	1998	Single institution	3.6	1° Diagnosis: total costs 2° Diagnosis: ordinary least squares	6	3669	6288
Pakyz et al[45]	HO-CDI	2007	Multi-institution (n=45) University HealthSystem Consortium administrative data	11.1	Matching and ordinary least squares	5	27,160	32,105
Tabak et al[2]	HO-CDI	2008	CareFusion clinical research database	2.3	Propensity score match	>30	6117	6972

Abbreviations: HO-CDI, health care–onset CDI; LOS, length of stay; N/A, not available; USD, US dollars.
a Costs estimates per case as reported in the paper.
b Costs adjusted using the US Department of Labor Bureau of Labor Statistics Consumer Price Indexes of Medical Care. Prices: http://data.bls.gov/pdq/SurveyOutputServlet.
c Song and colleagues[43] reported costs as direct variable rather than total costs; therefore, cost was doubled to equal total costs.
d Used mean LOS and costs reported for 1° and 2° diagnoses; reported costs weighted by proportion of 1° and 2° diagnoses.

Differences in patient populations may also lead to variation in estimates of hospital costs caused by CDI. Failure to control for costs of surgery and specific underlying illnesses may have resulted in an overestimation of costs attributable to CDI in the studies of Lipp and colleagues[44] and Pakyz and colleagues.[45] O'Brien and colleagues[42] also included surgical patients in their study and assumed all costs for patients admitted with CDI were attributable to CDI, whereas in actuality, patients may have been admitted to the hospital for other factors in addition to CDI.[42] With regard to other special populations, Zilberberg and colleagues[46] looked at mechanically ventilated patients and Lagu and colleagues[47] studied patients with sepsis, and they calculated CDI-attributable costs to be $13,293 and $5,251, respectively.

In nonsurgical patients, length of stay (LOS) is the major driver of hospital costs. Most studies report an attributable LOS of 2.3 to 5.5 days, with some reporting attributable LOS as high as 11.1 to 12.0 days.[2,7,8,34,42–45] The earlier discussion regarding the impact of methodological issues on cost estimates also pertains to attributable LOS estimates. Studies that used propensity score matching and controlled for a greater number of covariates had more conservative LOS estimates. Of the studies that adjusted for the greatest number of covariates, Dubberke and colleagues[7] and Tabak and colleagues[2] calculated similar attributable LOS caused by CDI of 2.8 and 2.3 days, respectively.

From the studies that reported attributable costs for all cases of in-hospital CDI, regardless of the method of cost adjustment, cost ranges from $3427 to $16,307.[7,8,42,43] Extrapolating from these estimates, based on the total number of discharges (362,510) from 2012 HCUP data, the total annual US acute care cost attributable to CDI is estimated to be $1.2 to $5.9 billion.[7,8,42,43,48]

After the initial episode of CDI, recurrent CDI results in further costs to the health care system. Hospital-level data indicate that approximately 15% of patients with the diagnosis of CDI are readmitted with recurrent CDI within 30 to 60 days after the initial episode.[7] McFarland[24] noted that patients may experience up to 14 episodes of CDI and require multiple hospitalizations, with a mean direct cost of medical care of $19,945 (2012 USD) for all episodes of CDI. In a large, retrospective cohort study limited to hospital costs of patients with CDI followed for 180 days, the attributable cost of recurrent CDI was estimated to be $12,425 (2012 USD).[49]

There are other potential costs attributable to CDI that are difficult to quantify. There may be lost opportunity for the hospital to generate revenue, as patients with CDI, who may incur a longer LOS, are placed in private rooms in most US hospitals. Patients with CDI contribute to the transmission of *C difficile* within the hospital, thereby perpetuating CDI and associated costs. Additionally, health care–onset CDI may soon be targeted by the Centers for Medicare and Medicaid Services as a nonreimbursable diagnosis, which has further implications for costs associated with CDI in the United States. Most of the available literature on the costs associated with CDI focuses on hospital facility costs and does not include those incurred in the outpatient setting, provider costs, or the indirect patient expenses associated with CDI. To the authors' knowledge, there are no data on costs to treat patients in LTCFs or in the community. In addition, there may be additional costs attributable to CDI, including lost time from work, costs related to increased transfers to LTCFs, additional testing, and costs of home health care. Hence, it is likely that the reported costs of CDI are grossly underestimated; therefore, CDI is a greater economic burden than is described in literature.

SUMMARY

CDI is a major cause of morbidity and mortality and contributor to health care costs. As CDI has emerged as the most common cause of HAIs in the United States, the future impact of CDI will likely continue to grow.[10] There is a significant need for a continued multidisciplinary approach to the prevention, treatment, reduction of recurrences, and control of spread of CDI.

REFERENCES

1. Dallal RM, Harbrecht BG, Boujoukas AJ, et al. Fulminant Clostridium difficile: an underappreciated and increasing cause of death and complications. Ann Surg 2002;235:363–72.
2. Tabak YP, Zilberberg MD, Johannes RS, et al. Attributable burden of hospital-onset Clostridium difficile infection: a propensity score matching study. Infect Control Hosp Epidemiol 2013;34:588–96.
3. Dubberke ER, Butler AM, Reske KA, et al. Attributable outcomes of endemic Clostridium difficile-associated disease in nonsurgical patients. Emerg Infect Dis 2008;14:1031–8.
4. Miller MA, Hyland M, Ofner-Agostini M, et al. Morbidity, mortality, and healthcare burden of nosocomial Clostridium difficile-associated diarrhea in Canadian hospitals. Infect Control Hosp Epidemiol 2002;23:137–40.
5. Loo VG, Poirier L, Miller MA, et al. A predominantly clonal multi-institutional outbreak of Clostridium difficile-associated diarrhea with high morbidity and mortality. N Engl J Med 2005;353:2442–9.
6. Gravel D, Miller M, Simor A, et al. Health care-associated Clostridium difficile infection in adults admitted to acute care hospitals in Canada: a Canadian Nosocomial Infection Surveillance Program Study. Clin Infect Dis 2009;48: 568–76.
7. Dubberke ER, Reske KA, Olsen MA, et al. Short- and long-term attributable costs of Clostridium difficile-associated disease in nonsurgical inpatients. Clin Infect Dis 2008;46:497–504.
8. Stewart DB, Hollenbeak CS. Clostridium difficile colitis: factors associated with outcome and assessment of mortality at a national level. J Gastrointest Surg 2011;15:1548–55.
9. Magill SS, Edwards JR, Bamberg W, et al. Multistate point-prevalence survey of health care-associated infections. N Engl J Med 2014;370:1198–208.
10. Miller BA, Chen LF, Sexton DJ, et al. Comparison of the burdens of hospital-onset, healthcare facility-associated Clostridium difficile infection and of healthcare-associated infection due to methicillin-resistant Staphylococcus aureus in community hospitals. Infect Control Hosp Epidemiol 2011;32:387–90.
11. Pepin J, Valiquette L, Gagnon S, et al. Outcomes of Clostridium difficile-associated disease treated with metronidazole or vancomycin before and after the emergence of NAP1/027. Am J Gastroenterol 2007;102:2781–8.
12. Muto CA, Pokrywka M, Shutt K, et al. A large outbreak of Clostridium difficile-associated disease with an unexpected proportion of deaths and colectomies at a teaching hospital following increased fluoroquinolone use. Infect Control Hosp Epidemiol 2005;26:273–80.
13. Dudukgian H, Sie E, Gonzalez-Ruiz C, et al. C. difficile colitis–predictors of fatal outcome. J Gastrointest Surg 2010;14:315–22.
14. Al-Abed YA, Gray EA, Rothnie ND. Outcomes of emergency colectomy for fulminant Clostridium difficile colitis. Surgeon 2010;8:330–3.
15. Pepin J, Valiquette L, Alary ME, et al. Clostridium difficile-associated diarrhea in a region of Quebec from 1991 to 2003: a changing pattern of disease severity. CMAJ 2004;171:466–72.

16. McDonald LC, Killgore GE, Thompson A, et al. An epidemic, toxin gene-variant strain of Clostridium difficile. N Engl J Med 2005;353:2433–41.
17. Kasper AM, Nyazee HA, Yokoe DS, et al. A multicenter study of Clostridium difficile infection-related colectomy, 2000-2006. Infect Control Hosp Epidemiol 2012;33:470–6.
18. Gash K, Brown E, Pullyblank A. Emergency subtotal colectomy for fulminant Clostridium difficile colitis - is a surgical solution considered for all patients? Ann R Coll Surg Engl 2010;92:56–60.
19. Rodriguez-Pardo D, Almirante B, Bartolome RM, et al. Epidemiology of Clostridium difficile infection and risk factors for unfavorable clinical outcomes: results of a hospital-based study in Barcelona, Spain. J Clin Microbiol 2013;51:1465–73.
20. Halabi WJ, Nguyen VQ, Carmichael JC, et al. Clostridium Difficile Colitis in the United States: a decade of trends, outcomes, risk factors for colectomy, and mortality after colectomy. J Am Coll Surg 2013;217:802–12.
21. See I, Mu Y, Cohen J, et al. NAP1 strain type predicts outcomes from Clostridium difficile infection. Clin Infect Dis 2014;58:1394–400.
22. Dallas KB, Condren A, Divino CM. Life after colectomy for fulminant Clostridium difficile colitis: a 7-year follow up study. Am J Surg 2014;207:533–9.
23. Garey KW, Sethi S, Yadav Y, et al. Meta-analysis to assess risk factors for recurrent Clostridium difficile infection. J Hosp Infect 2008;70:298–304.
24. McFarland LV, Surawicz CM, Rubin MS, et al. Recurrent *Clostridium difficile* disease: epidemiology and clinical characteristics. Infect Control Hosp Epidemiol 1999;20:43–9.
25. Fekety R, McFarland LV, Surawicz CM, et al. Recurrent Clostridium difficile diarrhea: characteristics of and risk factors for patients enrolled in a prospective, randomized, double-blinded trial. Clin Infect Dis 1997;24:324–33.
26. Pepin J, Alary ME, Valiquette L, et al. Increasing risk of relapse after treatment of Clostridium difficile colitis in Quebec, Canada. Clin Infect Dis 2005;40:1591–7.
27. McFarland LV. Alternative treatments for Clostridium difficile disease: what really works? J Med Microbiol 2005;54:101–11.
28. McFarland LV, Elmer GW, Surawicz CM. Breaking the cycle: treatment strategies for 163 cases of recurrent Clostridium difficile disease. Am J Gastroenterol 2002;97:1769–75.
29. Lessa FC. Incidence and insights into C. difficile infection epidemiology [abstract]. ID Week 2012. Available at: https://idsa.confex.com/idsa/2012/webprogram/Paper33395.html.
30. Elixhauser A, Steiner C, Gould C. Readmissions following hospitalizations with Clostridium difficile infections. Rockville (MD): Agency for Health Care Policy and Research; 2006-2012.
31. Micek ST, Schramm G, Morrow L, et al. Clostridium difficile infection: a multicenter study of epidemiology and outcomes in mechanically ventilated patients. Crit Care Med 2013;41:1968–75.
32. Centers for Disease Control and Prevention (CDC). Severe Clostridium difficile-associated disease in populations previously at low risk–four states, 2005. MMWR Morb Mortal Wkly Rep 2005;54:1201–5.
33. Chitnis AS, Holzbauer SM, Belflower RM, et al. Epidemiology of community-associated Clostridium difficile infection, 2009 through 2011. JAMA Intern Med 2013;173:1359–67.
34. Kyne L, Hamel MB, Polavaram R, et al. Health care costs and mortality associated with nosocomial diarrhea due to Clostridium difficile. Clin Infect Dis 2002;34:346–53.

35. Pepin J, Valiquette L, Cossette B. Mortality attributable to nosocomial Clostridium difficile-associated disease during an epidemic caused by a hypervirulent strain in Quebec. CMAJ 2005;173:1037–42.
36. Hall AJ, Curns AT, McDonald LC, et al. The roles of Clostridium difficile and norovirus among gastroenteritis-associated deaths in the United States, 1999-2007. Clin Infect Dis 2012;55:216–23.
37. Hoyert DL, Xu J. Deaths: preliminary data for 2011. Natl Vital Stat Rep 2012;61: 1–51.
38. Zilberberg MD, Shorr AF, Kollef MH. Increase in adult Clostridium difficile-related hospitalizations and case-fatality rate, United States, 2000-2005. Emerg Infect Dis 2008;14:929–31.
39. Walk ST, Micic D, Jain R, et al. Clostridium difficile ribotype does not predict severe infection. Clin Infect Dis 2012;55:1661–8.
40. Miller M, Gravel D, Mulvey M, et al. Health care-associated Clostridium difficile infection in Canada: patient age and infecting strain type are highly predictive of severe outcome and mortality. Clin Infect Dis 2010;50:194–201.
41. Walker AS, Eyre DW, Wylie DH, et al. Relationship between bacterial strain type, host biomarkers, and mortality in Clostridium difficile infection. Clin Infect Dis 2013;56(11):1589–600.
42. O'Brien JA, Lahue BJ, Caro JJ, et al. The emerging infectious challenge of clostridium difficile-associated disease in Massachusetts hospitals: clinical and economic consequences. Infect Control Hosp Epidemiol 2007;28:1219–27.
43. Song X, Bartlett JG, Speck K, et al. Rising economic impact of clostridium difficile-associated disease in adult hospitalized patient population. Infect Control Hosp Epidemiol 2008;29:823–8.
44. Lipp MJ, Nero DC, Callahan MA. Impact of hospital-acquired Clostridium difficile. J Gastroenterol Hepatol 2012;27:1733–7.
45. Pakyz A, Carroll NV, Harpe SE, et al. Economic impact of Clostridium difficile infection in a multihospital cohort of academic health centers. Pharmacotherapy 2011;31:546–51.
46. Zilberberg MD, Nathanson BH, Sadigov S, et al. Epidemiology and outcomes of clostridium difficile-associated disease among patients on prolonged acute mechanical ventilation. Chest 2009;136:752–8.
47. Lagu T, Stefan MS, Haessler S, et al. The impact of hospital-onset Clostridium difficile infection on outcomes of hospitalized patients with sepsis. J Hosp Med 2014;9:411–7.
48. HCUP National Inpatient Sample (NIS). Healthcare Cost and Utilization Project (HCUP) [report]. Rockville (MD): Agency for Healthcare Research and Quality; 2012. Available at: http://www.hcup-us.ahrq.gov/nisoverview.jsp. Accessed July 11, 2014.
49. Dubberke ER, Schaefer E, Reske KA, et al. Attributable inpatient costs of recurrent Clostridium difficile infections. Infect Control Hosp Epidemiol 2014;35: 1400–7.

The Potential of Probiotics to Prevent *Clostridium difficile* Infection

Stephen J. Allen, MB ChB, MRCP(UK) Paediatrics, DTM&H, MD

KEYWORDS

- *C difficile* diarrhea • Probiotic • Lactobacilli • *Bifidobacteria*
- *Saccharomyces boulardii*

KEY POINTS

- In this article, the familiar term probiotic is used for microbial preparations being evaluated in clinical trials rather than for organisms with a proven health benefit.
- Probiotics evaluated in the prevention of *Clostridium difficile* diarrhea (CDD) have included bacteria (mostly lactobacilli and *Bifidobacteria*) either as single strains or as blends of strains and/or species, in variable doses (number of organisms) and in variable formulations, and the yeast *Saccharomyces boulardii*.
- The interpretation of the findings of meta-analysis of probiotic trials is complicated by the difficulty in pooling results for different probiotic preparations. As a result, there is insufficient evidence to recommend the use of any specific probiotic preparation.
- The falling incidence of CDD among the older people in hospitals because of control measures complicates the further evaluation of probiotics for CDD prevention.

INTRODUCTION

C difficile has been the major cause of nosocomial infection in the hospital environment accounting for 15% to 39% of diarrhea that is associated with antibiotic treatment. Asymptomatic carriage results in new admissions constantly bringing *C difficile* into the hospital environment. The highly resistant nature of *C difficile* spores results in persistent contamination of the health care environment facilitating person-to-person spread by the fecal-oral route and requiring intensive control measures to prevent

Competing interests: The author has received research funding from Cultech Ltd, Port Talbot, UK; the Knowledge Exploitation Fund; Welsh Development Agency (project no. HE09 COL 1002); the National Ankylosing Spondylitis Society, UK; Yakult, UK; and the National Institute for Health Research Health Technology Assessment Programme (project numbers 06/39/02 and 08/13/24), UK. He was an invited guest at the Yakult Probiotic Symposium in 2011 and has received speaker's fees from Astellas Pharma, UK.
Department of Clinical Sciences, Liverpool School of Tropical Medicine, Pembroke Place, Liverpool L3 5QA, UK
E-mail address: stephen.allen@lstmed.ac.uk

Infect Dis Clin N Am 29 (2015) 135–144
http://dx.doi.org/10.1016/j.idc.2014.11.002
0891-5520/15/$ – see front matter © 2015 Elsevier Inc. All rights reserved.

id.theclinics.com

transmission. Although disease severity varies, CDD can be severe and complicated by toxic megacolon, intestinal perforation, and death.[1,2]

The 3 main risk factors for CDD, age greater than 65 years, admission to hospital, and exposure to antibiotics, have been recognized for many years.[1,2] A prospective study of adults (age >18 years) admitted to hospitals in Canada reported that increasing age, exposure to antibiotics, treatment with proton pump inhibitors (PPIs), and prior recent hospital admission predicted CDD.[3] A retrospective study of patients admitted to hospitals in Europe identified age greater than or equal to 65 years, severe comorbidity, and recent treatment with cephalosporins and amino-penicillin-β-lactamase inhibitor combinations as risk factors for CDD.[4] A large, randomized controlled trial of a probiotic in the prevention of CDD found that both increased age (>77 years) and longer duration of antibiotic treatment (>8 days) were associated with an increased risk of CDD.[5]

WHAT ARE PROBIOTICS?

Probiotics are defined as "live microbial organisms which, when administered in adequate numbers, are beneficial to health."[6] However, the term probiotic is used more generally in research studies for microbial preparations that are being evaluated for health benefits, and it is this broader meaning that is used here.

The characteristics of microbial strains classified as probiotics are listed in **Box 1**.[6,7] Organisms that have been evaluated for the prevention of CDD include single strains and blends of bacteria (*Lactobacillus* spp, *Bifidobacteria* spp, *Streptococcus thermophilus*) and the yeast *S boulardii* (not of human origin).[8]

Lactobacilli and *Bifidobacteria*, bacteria commonly used as probiotics, are generally regarded as safe by the Food and Agriculture Organization of the United Nations.[6] Probiotics have been administered without short-term adverse effects to many vulnerable groups of people, such as preterm infants and people with human immunodeficiency virus infection. Systematic reviews of trials of mainly single strains or mixtures of

---

Box 1
Characteristics of probiotic organisms

- Human origin
- Live
- Safe/non-pathogenic
- Resistant to gastric acid, bile, and pancreatic juice to survive transit through the gastrointestinal tract
- Able to withstand technological processes and remain viable during shelf life
- Induce a host response once ingested
- Result in a functional or clinical benefit to the host
- Characterized using phenotypic and genotypic techniques
- Deposited in an internationally recognized culture collection

(*Data from* Food and Agriculture Organization of the UN and WHO. Report of a joint FAO/WHO working group on drafting guidelines for the evaluation of probiotics in food. Geneva (Switzerland): World Health Organization; 2002. Available at: http://www.who.int/entity/foodsafety/fs_management/en/probiotic_guidelines.pdf. Accessed July 8, 2014; and Parkes GC, Sanderson JD, Whelan K. The mechanisms and efficacy of probiotics in the prevention of *Clostridium difficile*-associated diarrhoea. Lancet Infect Dis 2009;9:237–44.)

lactobacilli and *Bifidobacteria* administered to medium-risk and critically ill patients did not identify adverse events associated with these organisms.[9,10] However, lactic acid bacteria have caused occasional infections in immunocompromized people and those with artificial heart valves,[11] and the ongoing assessment of safety in clinical trials is recommended.[9]

WHY MIGHT PROBIOTICS BE EFFECTIVE IN PREVENTING *CLOSTRIDIUM DIFFICILE* DIARRHEA?

There are several stages in the progression from the initial colonization with *C difficile* to mild CDD through to severe disease in which probiotics may exert a preventive or ameliorative effect. Exposure to antibiotics, the most consistently established risk factor for CDD, has profound and diverse effects on both the composition and the function of the gut microbiome.[12] Although the exact pathogenic mechanisms whereby antibiotic treatment results in CDD are unknown and may differ with different antibiotics, 2 major mechanisms have been proposed (**Box 2**).

CDD is associated with the effects of the release of 2 exotoxins A and B, which increase the permeability of the colonic mucosa through impairment of tight junction integrity and also result in the acute necroinflammatory changes observed in pseudo-membranous colitis.[13] Several properties of probiotic organisms identified in vitro and in vivo may allow them to replenish the antibiotic-depleted gut flora to restore colonization resistance, and also enhance the integrity and barrier function of the gut epithelium, and therefore prevent or ameliorate CDD (**Box 3**).[14–17]

The particular mechanisms of action that are most important in the prevention of CDD and the degree to which these are shared widely among different probiotic organisms or are species or strain specific are unknown. In vitro studies have demonstrated that a range of microbes inhibit *C difficile*[18–20] and also reduce the inflammation caused by *C difficile* infection.[21] Both single strains and blends of strains and/or species have been studied with results indicating that mechanisms inhibiting *C difficile* and the associated inflammation are strain specific. However, despite attempts to replicate the complex, competitive environment of the distal colon, whether or not effects in vitro will translate to the clinical arena is uncertain.

Alongside the broad consensus that probiotic effects are strain specific, there is general agreement that blends of organisms are more effective than single strains in maintaining a beneficial gut microbiota.[22] In general, in both animal and human studies and across a range of health outcomes, blends of organisms rather than single strains tend to have greater efficacy.[23] The multiple stages in the progression from *C difficile* colonization to infection argue that a multistrain probiotic is likely to be more effective than a single-stain probiotic both in the prevention of disease and in nosocomial transmission.[17]

There is emerging evidence regarding differences in the composition of the gut microbiome in established CDD cases compared with non-CDD diarrhea controls and/or healthy individuals.[24,25] However, a greater understanding is needed regarding

---

Box 2
Mechanisms by which exposure to antibiotics results in CDD

- Depletion of the gut flora resulting in impaired colonization resistance to *C difficile*
- Exertion of stress on vegetative *C difficile* organisms resulting in exotoxin secretion and, thereby, mucosal inflammation

---

Box 3
Properties of probiotic organisms that may prevent or ameliorate CDD

- Enhanced colonization resistance
  - ○ Secretion of antimicrobial peptides to kill or inhibit pathogens
  - ○ Competition for nutrients
  - ○ Competition for attachment sites on intestinal mucus and epithelium
  - ○ Acidification of the gut contents by the production of lactic acid and other organic acids that inhibit pathogen growth
- Enhanced mucosal integrity and barrier function
  - ○ Increased secretion of mucus
  - ○ Enhanced integrity of tight junctions between epithelial cells
  - ○ Decreased epithelial cell apoptosis
  - ○ Increased secretory immunoglobulin A production
  - ○ Increased secretion of defensins and other antimicrobial peptides
- Downregulation of gene expression to decrease virulence and/or growth through quorum sensing
- Neutralization of *C difficile* toxins

Data from Refs.[14–17]

---

the characteristics of the gut microbiota that may be resistant to antibiotic treatment or the development of CDD after antibiotic exposure in advance of disease onset.[14] There are several factors that suggest that this will be challenging. The composition of the gut microbiome varies markedly between individuals,[26] varies to a greater degree in the elderly than in young people, and is affected by chronic disease, frailty, diet, residence, and care setting.[27] In addition, specific variations in microbiome composition may underlie susceptibility to *C difficile* colonization as opposed to disease and also colonization with different *C difficile* ribotypes.[25] Finally, rather than specific antibiotic treatment regimens, the risk of CDD seems to be associated with cumulative antibiotic exposure over time,[28] but the number of different antibiotics and duration of treatment required in individual patients is often difficult to predict at the start of therapy.

The very large number of different probiotics available and the uncertainty as to whether strain-specific effects demonstrated in vitro will translate in vivo makes the selection of probiotic preparations for evaluation in human trials challenging.

WHAT ARE THE FINDINGS FROM CLINICAL TRIALS?

A recent meta-analysis pooled the findings of 23 randomized controlled trials of 4213 children and adults that evaluated many different probiotics, including the yeast *S. boulardii*, in the prevention of CDD.[8] Overall, probiotics were found to markedly and significantly reduce the frequency of CDD (fixed-effects analysis; risk ratio 0.36; 95% confidence interval [CI] 0.26–0.49; **Fig. 1**). There was consistency in results across studies ($I^2 = 0.0$), and probiotics remained clinically effective in worst-case assumptions for missing outcome data. Similar effects of the probiotics were observed when studies in adults and children were compared. This meta-analysis updates the findings of previous meta-analyses.[29–32]

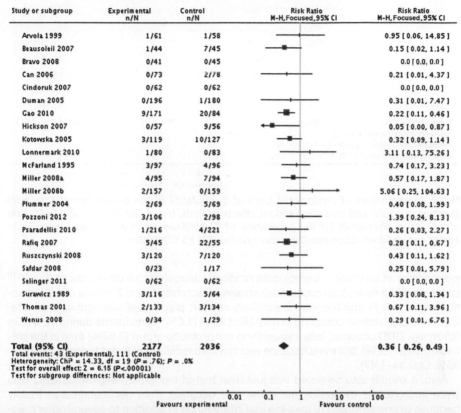

Study or subgroup	Experimental n/N	Control n/N	Risk Ratio M-H,Focused,95% CI	Risk Ratio M-H,Focused,95% CI
Arvola 1999	1/61	1/58		0.95 [0.06, 14.85]
Beausoleil 2007	1/44	7/45		0.15 [0.02, 1.14]
Bravo 2008	0/41	0/45		0.0 [0.0, 0.0]
Can 2006	0/73	2/78		0.21 [0.01, 4.37]
Cindoruk 2007	0/62	0/62		0.0 [0.0, 0.0]
Duman 2005	0/196	1/180		0.31 [0.01, 7.47]
Gao 2010	9/171	20/84		0.22 [0.11, 0.46]
Hickson 2007	0/57	9/56		0.05 [0.00, 0.87]
Kotowska 2005	3/119	10/127		0.32 [0.09, 1.14]
Lonnermark 2010	1/80	0/83		3.11 [0.13, 75.26]
McFarland 1995	3/97	4/96		0.74 [0.17, 3.23]
Miller 2008a	4/95	7/94		0.57 [0.17, 1.87]
Miller 2008b	2/157	0/159		5.06 [0.25, 104.63]
Plummer 2004	2/69	5/69		0.40 [0.08, 1.99]
Pozzoni 2012	3/106	2/98		1.39 [0.24, 8.13]
Psaradellis 2010	1/216	4/221		0.26 [0.03, 2.27]
Rafiq 2007	5/45	22/55		0.28 [0.11, 0.67]
Ruszczynski 2008	3/120	7/120		0.43 [0.11, 1.62]
Safdar 2008	0/23	1/17		0.25 [0.01, 5.79]
Selinger 2011	0/62	0/62		0.0 [0.0, 0.0]
Surawicz 1989	3/116	5/64		0.33 [0.08, 1.34]
Thomas 2001	2/133	3/134		0.67 [0.11, 3.96]
Wenus 2008	0/34	1/29		0.29 [0.01, 6.76]
Total (95% CI)	**2177**	**2036**		**0.36 [0.26, 0.49]**

Total events: 43 (Experimental), 111 (Control)
Heterogeneity: Chi² = 14.33, df = 19 (P = .76); P = .0%
Test for overall effect: Z = 6.15 (P<.00001)
Test for subgroup differences: Not applicable

0.01   0.1   1   10   100
Favours experimental   Favours control

Fig. 1. Meta-analysis of randomized trials of probiotics in the prevention of *C difficile* diarrhea in adults and children; fixed-effects analysis. (*From* Goldenberg JZ, Ma SS, Saxton JD, et al. Probiotics for the prevention of *Clostridium difficile*-associated diarrhea in adults and children. Cochrane Database Syst Rev 2013;5:CD006095.)

Subgroup analysis was performed for specific probiotic species. Where the findings from 2 or more studies were pooled, efficacy remained statistically significant for the yeast *S. boulardii* (**Fig. 2**) and a blend of *Lactobacillus acidophilus* and *Lactobacillus casei* (**Fig. 3**), but not for *Lactobacillus* GG (random-effects model, risk ratio 0.63; 95% CI 0.30–1.33).

Despite the apparently encouraging findings, only 3 of the included trials reported a statistically significant effect of the probiotic (see **Fig. 1**). In 2 of these trials, the frequency of CDD was unusually high in the control group (20/84, 23.8%[33] and 22/55, 40.0%; Rafiq, unpublished data, 2007). Also, research methods and reporting were assessed to be poor in many of the studies included in the review. Therefore, caution is needed in the interpretation of the findings and also in generalizing the effect of probiotics to specific settings.

A recent large UK study, although reporting findings consistent with this meta-analysis, did not demonstrate a statistically significant effect of a probiotic in the prevention of CDD.[34] The PLACIDE (Probiotic lactobacilli and bifidobacteria in antibiotic-associated diarrhoea and *Clostridium difficile* diarrhoea in the elderly) study recruited almost 3000 older (≥65 years) people exposed to antibiotics and admitted to 1 of 5 hospitals in 2 geographically distant regions. Potential risk factors for CDD

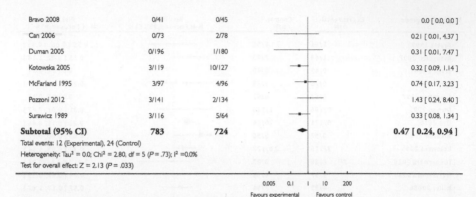

Bravo 2008	0/41	0/45		0.0 [0.0, 0.0]
Can 2006	0/73	2/78		0.21 [0.01, 4.37]
Duman 2005	0/196	1/180		0.31 [0.01, 7.47]
Kotowska 2005	3/119	10/127		0.32 [0.09, 1.14]
McFarland 1995	3/97	4/96		0.74 [0.17, 3.23]
Pozzoni 2012	3/141	2/134		1.43 [0.24, 8.40]
Surawicz 1989	3/116	5/64		0.33 [0.08, 1.34]
Subtotal (95% CI)	**783**	**724**		**0.47 [0.24, 0.94]**

Total events: 12 (Experimental), 24 (Control)
Heterogeneity: Tau² = 0.0; Chi² = 2.80, df = 5 (P = .73); I² =0.0%
Test for overall effect: Z = 2.13 (P = .033)

0.005   0.1   1   10   200
Favours experimental   Favours control

Fig. 2. Meta-analysis of randomized trials of *S. boulardii* in the prevention of *C difficile* diarrhea in adults and children; random-effects analysis. (*From* Goldenberg JZ, Ma SS, Saxton JD, et al. Probiotics for the prevention of *Clostridium difficile*-associated diarrhea in adults and children. Cochrane Database Syst Rev 2013;5:CD006095.)

were similar at baseline in participants randomly allocated to a daily dose of 6×10^{10} organisms of a multistrain probiotic (2 strains of lactobacilli and 2 strains of *Bifidobacteria*) for 21 days and those who received an inert placebo of identical appearance. CDD was uncommon occurring in only 29 of 2941 (1.0%) participants during 12 weeks follow-up. CDD occurred less frequently in the probiotic group (0.82%) than in the placebo group (1.2%), but the difference was not statistically significant (relative risk 0.71; 95% CI 0.34–1.47).

Also, it should also be noted that just over half of the 17,420 eligible patients who were approached to participate in the trial declined. This declination was mainly because of unwillingness to take the trial intervention in addition to several other medications for comorbid illnesses that these people were already taking. These investigators recommended that these practical issues need to be considered in any future trials undertaken in similar populations.[34]

Only one other clinical trial has reported outcomes specifically in patients aged 65 years or older.[35] A blend of 2 *Lactobacillus* spp and *S. thermophilus* compared with placebo reduced CDD (0/56, 0% vs 9/53, 17.0%). However, patients were highly selected[36] and the relatively high frequency of CDD in the placebo group is not typical of many health care settings.

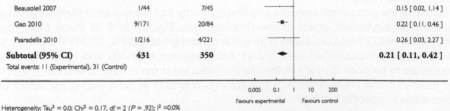

Beausoleil 2007	1/44	7/45		0.15 [0.02, 1.14]
Gao 2010	9/171	20/84		0.22 [0.11, 0.46]
Psaradellis 2010	1/216	4/221		0.26 [0.03, 2.27]
Subtotal (95% CI)	**431**	**350**		**0.21 [0.11, 0.42]**

Total events: 11 (Experimental), 31 (Control)

0.005   0.1   1   10   200
Favours experimental   Favours control

Heterogeneity: Tau² = 0.0; Chi² = 0.17, df = 2 (P = .92); I² =0.0%
Test for overall effect: Z = 4.54 (P<.00001)

Fig. 3. Meta-analysis of randomized trials of a blend of *L. acidophilus* and *L. casei* in the prevention of *C difficile* diarrhea in adults and children; random-effects analysis. (*From* Goldenberg JZ, Ma SS, Saxton JD, et al. Probiotics for the prevention of *Clostridium difficile*-associated diarrhea in adults and children. Cochrane Database Syst Rev 2013;5:CD006095.)

SUMMARY AND DISCUSSION

Whether or not probiotics have a role in the prevention of CDD remains unclear. Despite numerous clinical trials, meta-analysis is undermined by many small and poor-quality studies and the uncertainty regarding species and strain-specific effects, which question the validity of pooling results across studies that have evaluated different probiotics. The difficulty in the interpretation of findings from meta-analysis of probiotic trials has been highlighted, and an approach has been proposed to assist clinicians in evaluating the strength of the evidence for specific probiotic strains.[37]

In addition, the recent PLACIDE study did not show clear evidence of probiotic effectiveness despite using a high-dose, multistrain probiotic that included lactobacilli and *Bifidobacteria*.[34] This lack of a clear effectiveness of the probiotic in the largest clinical trial of a probiotic ever reported, which apparently adopted sound research methodology,[38] casts doubt on the validity of this approach for the prevention of CDD.

Although the development of clinical practice guidelines will require more robust data from high-quality clinical trials that recruit sufficient patients to give a clear result, a major challenge in designing future clinical trials is the almost infinite number of different strains and blends of microbial preparations and treatment regimens that could be evaluated. Key issues to address will be single strain versus blends of strains and/or species, dose (ie, number of organisms), duration of administration, and vehicle for delivery. Perhaps most importantly, the selection of microbial interventions for evaluation in future clinical trials will require a better understanding of the disease mechanisms underlying CDD. The critical question is what specific disease mechanism might a specific probiotic address? The practical limitations of administering an additional intervention in the most susceptible patients, ie, older hospitalized people likely already to be taking several medications, also needs to be considered.[34]

Finally, the falling incidence of CDD among older hospitalized patients in the United Kingdom and similar settings in recent years, as a result of concerted efforts at improved prevention of health-care-acquired infections,[5,39–41] indicates that future clinical trials may have to be targeted at high-risk groups; these include patients exposed to specific antibiotics or with additional potential risk factors such as PPI therapy.[42] If a high-risk population cannot be readily identified, the advent of potentially highly effective treatments such as fecal transplant (discussed in this issue by Young and Rao) may mean that further probiotic trials for the prevention of CDD will need careful justification.

REFERENCES

1. Viswanathan VK, Mallozzi MJ, Vedantam G. *Clostridium difficile* infection: an overview of the disease and its pathogenesis, epidemiology and interventions. Gut Microbes 2010;1:234–42.
2. Dubberke ER, Haslam DB, Lanzas C, et al. The ecology and pathobiology of *Clostridium difficile* infections: an interdisciplinary challenge. Zoonoses Public Health 2011;58:4–20.
3. Loo VG, Bourgault AM, Poirier L, et al. Host and pathogen factors for *Clostridium difficile* infection and colonization. N Engl J Med 2011;365:1693–703.
4. Bauer MP, Notermans DW, van Benthem BH, et al. *Clostridium difficile* infection in Europe: a hospital-based survey. Lancet 2011;377:63–73.
5. Allen SJ, Wareham K, Wang D, et al. A high-dose preparation of lactobacilli and *Bifidobacteria* in the prevention of antibiotic-associated and *Clostridium difficile* diarrhoea in older people admitted to hospital: a multicentre, randomised,

double-blind, placebo-controlled, parallel arm trial (PLACIDE). Health Technol Assess 2013;17:1–140.

6. Food and Agriculture Organization of the UN and WHO. Report of a joint FAO/WHO working group on drafting guidelines for the evaluation of probiotics in food. Geneva (Switzerland): World Health Organization; 2002. Available at: http://www. who.int/entity/foodsafety/fs_management/en/probiotic_guidelines.pdf. Accessed July 8, 2014.

7. Parkes GC, Sanderson JD, Whelan K. The mechanisms and efficacy of probiotics in the prevention of *Clostridium difficile*-associated diarrhoea. Lancet Infect Dis 2009;9:237–44.

8. Goldenberg JZ, Ma SS, Saxton JD, et al. Probiotics for the prevention of *Clostridium difficile*-associated diarrhea in adults and children. Cochrane Database Syst Rev 2013;(5):CD006095.

9. Hempel S, Newberry S, Ruelaz A, et al. Safety of probiotics used to reduce risk and prevent or treat disease. Evid Rep Technol Assess (Full Rep) 2011;200: 1–645.

10. Whelan K, Myers CE. Safety of probiotics in patients receiving nutritional support: a systematic review of case reports, randomized controlled trials, and nonrandomized trials. Am J Clin Nutr 2010;91:687–703.

11. Hammerman C, Bin-Nun A, Kaplan M. Safety of probiotics: comparison of two popular strains. BMJ 2006;333:1006–8.

12. Antunes LC, Han J, Ferreira RB, et al. Effect of antibiotic treatment on the intestinal metabolome. Antimicrob Agents Chemother 2011;55:1494–503.

13. Pothoulakis C, Lamont JT. Microbes and microbial toxins: paradigms for microbial-mucosal interactions II. The integrated response of the intestine to *Clostridium difficile* toxins. Am J Physiol Gastrointest Liver Physiol 2001;280: G178–83.

14. Britton RA, Young VB. Role of the intestinal microbiota in resistance to colonization by *Clostridium difficile*. Gastroenterology 2014;146:1547–53.

15. Plummer S, Weaver MA, Harris JC, et al. *Clostridium difficile* pilot study: effects of probiotic supplementation on the incidence of *C. difficile* diarrhoea. Int Microbiol 2004;7:59–62.

16. Ohland CL, Macnaughton WK. Probiotic bacteria and intestinal epithelial barrier function. Am J Physiol Gastrointest Liver Physiol 2010;298:G807–19.

17. Hell M, Bernhofer C, Stalzer P, et al. Probiotics in *Clostridium difficile* infection: reviewing the need for a multistrain probiotic. Benef Microbes 2013;4:39–51.

18. Naaber P, Smidt I, Stsepetova J, et al. Inhibition of *Clostridium difficile* strains by intestinal *Lactobacillus* species. J Med Microbiol 2004;53:551–4.

19. Tejero-Sariñena S, Barlow J, Costabile A, et al. Antipathogenic activity of probiotics against Salmonella Typhimurium and *Clostridium difficile* in anaerobic batch culture systems: is it due to synergies in probiotic mixtures or the specificity of single strains? Anaerobe 2013;24:60–5.

20. Schoster A, Kokotovic B, Permin A, et al. In vitro inhibition of *Clostridium difficile* and *Clostridium perfringens* by commercial probiotic strains. Anaerobe 2013;20: 36–41.

21. Boonma P, Spinler JK, Venable SF, et al. *Lactobacillus rhamnosus* L34 and *Lactobacillus casei* L39 suppress *Clostridium difficile*-induced IL-8 production by colonic epithelial cells. BMC Microbiol 2014;14:177.

22. Chapman CM, Gibson GR, Rowland I. Health benefits of probiotics: are mixtures more effective than single strains? Eur J Nutr 2011;50:1–17.

23. Timmerman HM, Koning CJ, Mulder L, et al. Monostrain, multistrain and multispecies probiotics – a comparison of functionality and efficacy. Int J Food Microbiol 2004;96:219–33.
24. Schubert AM, Rogers MA, Ring C, et al. Microbiome data distinguish patients with *Clostridium difficile* infection and non-*C. difficile*-associated diarrhea from healthy controls. MBio 2014;5. e01021–14.
25. Skraban J, Dzeroski S, Zenko B, et al. Gut microbiota patterns associated with colonization of different *Clostridium difficile* ribotypes. PLoS One 2013;8:e58005.
26. Arumugam M, Raes J, Pelletier E, et al. Enterotypes of the human gut microbiome. Nature 2011;473:174–80.
27. Claesson MJ, Cusack S, O' Sullivan O, et al. Composition, variability, and temporal stability of the intestinal microbiota of the elderly. Proc Natl Acad Sci U S A 2011;108(Suppl 1):4586–91.
28. Stevens V, Dumyati G, Fine LS, et al. Cumulative antibiotic exposures over time and the risk of *Clostridium difficile* infection. Clin Infect Dis 2011;53:42–8.
29. Hempel S, Newberry SJ, Maher AR, et al. Probiotics for the prevention and treatment of antibiotic-associated diarrhea: a systematic review and meta-analysis. JAMA 2012;307:1959–69.
30. Dendukuri N, Costa V, McGregor M, et al. Probiotic therapy for the prevention and treatment of *Clostridium difficile* -associated diarrhea: a systematic review. CMAJ 2005;173:167–70.
31. Johnston BC, Ma SS, Goldenberg JZ, et al. Probiotics for the Prevention of *Clostridium difficile*– associated diarrhea: a systematic review and meta-analysis. Ann Intern Med 2012;18:878–88.
32. Hickson M. Probiotics in the prevention of antibiotic-associated diarrhoea and *Clostridium difficile* infection. Therap Adv Gastroenterol 2011;4:185–97.
33. Gao XW, Mubasher M, Fang CY, et al. Dose-response efficacy of a proprietary probiotic formula of *Lactobacillus acidophilus* CL1285 and *Lactobacillus casei* LBC80R for antibiotic-associated diarrhea and *Clostridium difficile*-associated diarrhea prophylaxis in adult patients. Am J Gastroenterol 2010;105:1636–41.
34. Allen SJ, Wareham K, Wang D, et al. Lactobacilli and *Bifidobacteria* in the prevention of antibiotic-associated diarrhoea and *Clostridium difficile* diarrhoea in older inpatients (PLACIDE): a randomised, double-blind, placebo-controlled, multicentre trial. Lancet 2013;382:1249–57.
35. Hickson M, D'Souza AL, Muthu N, et al. Use of probiotic *Lactobacillus* preparation to prevent diarrhoea associated with antibiotics: randomised double blind placebo controlled trial. BMJ 2007;335:80.
36. McFarland LV. Diarrhoea associated with antibiotic use. BMJ 2007;335:54–5.
37. McFarland LV. Deciphering meta-analytic results: a mini-review of probiotics for the prevention of paediatric antibiotic-associated diarrhoea and *Clostridium difficile* infections. Benef Microbes 2014;1–6. http://dx.doi.org/10.3920/BM2014.0034. Accessed July 9, 2014.
38. Ziakas PD, Mylonakis E. Probiotics did not prevent antibiotic-associated or *C. difficile* diarrhea in hospitalized older patients. Ann Intern Med 2014;160:JC6.
39. Health Protection Agency. Results from the mandatory *Clostridium difficile* reporting scheme. 2013. Available at: http://www.hpa.org.uk/Topics/InfectiousDiseases/InfectionsAZ/ClostridiumDifficile/EpidemiologicalData/MandatorySurveillance/cdiff MandatoryReportingScheme/. Accessed July 10, 2014.

40. Public Health Wales. All Wales Commentaries: *Clostridium difficile* reports. 2012. Available at: http://www.wales.nhs.uk/sites3/page.cfm?orgid=379&pid=18490. Accessed July 10, 2014.

41. Kanerva M, Mentula S, Virolainen-Julkunen A, et al. Reduction in *Clostridium difficile* infections in Finland, 2008-2010. J Hosp Infect 2013;83:127–31.

42. Janarthanan S, Ditah I, Adler DG, et al. *Clostridium difficile*-associated diarrhea and proton pump inhibitor therapy: a meta-analysis. Am J Gastroenterol 2012; 107:1001–10.

The Prospect for Vaccines to Prevent *Clostridium difficile* Infection

Chandrabali Ghose, PhD[a],*, Ciarán P. Kelly, MD[b]

KEYWORDS

- *Clostridium difficile* • Infection • Vaccinations • Passive immunotherapy

KEY POINTS

- The pathogenicity of *Clostridium difficile* is primarily mediated through the release of 2 toxins: toxin A (TcdA) and toxin B (TcdB).
- The incidence and severity of *Clostridium difficile* infection (CDI) have risen dramatically since the turn of the century, leading to increased CDI-related morbidity, mortality, and economic costs.
- Novel approaches are sorely needed to stop the CDI epidemic. Efficacious prophylactic and therapeutic vaccines against *C difficile* are very likely to be cost-effective based on computer-simulation models and are an attractive approach to stem the spread of CDI.
- Innate immune defense mechanisms against CDI include the host's normal microbiota and the mucosal immune system that includes the intestinal epithelial cells.
- Although fewer than 5% of adults and older children are colonized, antibodies against *C difficile* are present in many adults and older children because of transient exposure to *C difficile* at infancy or from repeated exposure in adulthood from the environment.
- Antibody responses to *C difficile* TcdA and TcdB appear to be protective against primary disease and against recurrence.
- Given the importance of the humoral response against toxins, passive administration of neutralizing antitoxin antibodies could provide both a preventative and a therapeutic passive immunization strategy.
- Although a strong immune response against TcdA and TcdB may prevent the development of CDI, it does not prevent colonization of the host by the bacterium. Therefore, surface proteins involved in adherence, such as S-layer proteins, flagellar proteins, FliC and FliD, protease Cwp84, the Fbp68 fibronectin binding protein, and the GroEl heat-shock protein, have been studied as potential vaccine candidates in animals. Vaccines targeting nontoxin antigens will likely be needed to prevent colonization, reduce spore production, and interrupt disease transmission.

[a] Aaron Diamond AIDS Research Center, 455 First Avenue, 7th Floor, New York, NY 10016, USA;
[b] Division of Gastroenterology, Beth Israel Deaconess Medical Center, Harvard Medical School, 330 Brookline Avenue, Boston, MA 02215, USA
* Corresponding author.
E-mail address: cghose@adarc.org

Infect Dis Clin N Am 29 (2015) 145–162
http://dx.doi.org/10.1016/j.idc.2014.11.013
0891-5520/15/$ – see front matter © 2015 Elsevier Inc. All rights reserved.

id.theclinics.com

INTRODUCTION
Clostridium difficile Infection

Clostridium difficile is a spore-forming gram-positive organism that is the leading cause of nosocomial antibiotic-associated infectious diarrhea, commonly known as *C difficile* infection (CDI).[1] Broad-spectrum antibiotic usage (such as fluoroquinolones, second-generation and third-generation cephalosporines and clindamycin), hospitalization, age greater than 65 years, and severe underlying disease each increase the risk of developing CDI. Symptoms range from asymptomatic intestinal colonization to diarrhea, colitis, pseudomembranous colitis, and death.[2] Colonization resistance in the form of direct microbe-microbe interactions in the gut, competition for the same niche and nutrients, and the production of antimicrobial molecules usually prevent ingested *C difficile* from establishing an infection. The perturbation and elimination of the healthy microflora of the gut following the use of broad-spectrum antibiotics lead to the loss of colonization resistance, allowing *C difficile* spores to germinate, colonize, replicate, and produce adequate levels of toxins to cause disease. In addition to changes in the gut microbial community, antibiotic treatment induces substantial changes in the gut metabolome, leading to changes in the level of bile acids, especially taurocholate, which is essential for *C difficile* spore germination.[3,4]

The pathogenicity of *C difficile* is mediated primarily through the release of 2 toxins: toxin A (TcdA) and toxin B (TcdB).[5] The toxin genes as well as genes involved in the regulation of toxin production (sigma factor, TcdR, and putative anti-sigma factors, TcdC) as well as TcdE (a holinlike protein thought to facilitate toxin release across the bacterial cell membrane) are each present on the 19.6-kb pathogenicity locus (PaloC) of *C difficile*.[6] Both of the large protein exotoxins (TcdA, 308 kDa; TcdB, 270 kDa) function as glucosyltransferases that inactivate Rho, Rac, and Cdc42 within eukaryotic target cells, leading to actin polymerization, opening of tight junctions, and ultimately, cell death.[7] The toxins have 4 functional domains consisting of an N-terminal glucosyltransferase domain, an endopeptidase domain, a membrane translocation section, and a C-terminal receptor-binding domain (RBD) consisting of repeating units of 21, 30, or 50 amino acid residues.[8,9] Although the receptors for these toxins have not been identified, the crystal structure for the RBD of TcdA has been resolved.[10–12] The 1.85-A resolution crystal structure reveals a β-solenoid fold containing 32 small repeats of 15 to 21 residues and 7 large repeats of 30 residues. The RBD of TcdB is thought to be similar to TcdA, although structural data are unavailable. Following receptor binding and endocytosis, the toxins translocate through the early endosomal compartments into the cytosol.[13] The toxins are processed by autocatalytic cleavage in the endosomal compartments, such that only the N-terminal enzymatic domain is released into the cytosol.[9] In the cytosol, the small GTPases are glucosylated, thus deregulating downstream signal transduction pathways, leading ultimately to cell death. Previously, it was thought that TcdA initiated intestinal epithelial damage and mucosal disruption that allowed TcdB to gain access to underlying cells, but recent studies using TcdA-negative *C difficile* mutants demonstrate the importance of TcdB in a CDI animal model. There have also been numerous reports of TcdA-negative/TcdB-positive strains of *C difficile* isolated from patients with CDI and colitis.[14,15] There have been no substantiated reports of TcdA-positive/TcdB-negative strains. Although the toxins are essential for symptomatic disease, their role in colonization is unknown. *C difficile* has been shown to preferentially bind the basolateral surface of epithelial cells. Sublethal concentration of TcdA has recently been shown to alter cell polarity, allowing *C difficile* to gain access to basolateral receptors needed for successful colonization of colonic mucosa, suggesting a role for the toxins in colonization.[16] Non-toxin-producing *C difficile* strains account for about 20% of circulating strains and do not cause CDI.

The Changing Epidemiology of Clostridium difficile Infection in the Twenty-first Century

The last decade has seen a dramatic change in the epidemiology of CDI. Once an easily treated bacterial infection in the elderly, associated with antibiotic use and prolonged stays at the hospital, CDI has now evolved into an epidemic that is associated with a high rate of mortality, causing disease in patients thought to be considered low risk.[17] Outbreaks of CDI associated with increased severity were first reported in the United States and Canada between 2000 and 2003 with mortality rates reaching 13.7% compared with 4.7% from a decade earlier.[18] Large outbreaks in one UK hospital demonstrated the severity of the disease: 33 of 334 patients died of CDI acquired during 2 outbreaks in 2003 and 2005.[19] Outbreaks with high mortality have since been reported in mainland Europe, Central America, followed by Asia, Australia, and South America. The changing epidemiology of CDI is partly due to the emergence of a hypervirulent strain of *C difficile* identified as polymerase chain reaction ribotype 027, North American pulse field type 1, or restriction endonuclease analysis group B1, commonly known as BI/NAP1/027. *C difficile* has now replaced methicillin-resistant *Staphylococcus aureus* as the leading cause of fatal nosocomial infections and is the cause of 14,000 deaths a year in the United States alone.[20]

The changing epidemiology is also characterized by community-acquired CDI, in younger, healthy individuals considered to be at low risk, with no previous exposure to antibiotics. Large-scale surveillance data suggest that approximately 20% or greater of all CDI cases are community associated. In addition, *C difficile* is now an endemic problem in certain areas, suggesting a source or a reservoir of CDIs not associated with symptomatic patients.[21] Peripartum women, health care and laboratory workers, and children as young as 19 months have been infected with hypervirulent *C difficile* BI/NAP1/027 strains, causing rapid changes in the diagnosis and treatment of these population groups presenting with diarrhea.[22]

Although epidemic *C difficile* BI/NAP1/027 has been associated with more severe disease, the reason for the heightened virulence is still unknown. Extensive analysis of the genes present on PaloC of these hypervirulent strains initially showed that these strains produced more toxins, possibly because of deletions present in the negative regulator *tcdC*, although further studies revealed that the 18-bp deletion did not have any effect on toxin production.[23] Lanis and colleagues[24] showed that TcdB from the epidemic BI/NAP1/027 strain of *C difficile* was more likely to be lethal, caused more extensive brain hemorrhage, and was antigenically variable compared with TcdB produced by a reference strain.

In addition to TcdA and TcdB, hypervirulent *C difficile* strains express an iotalike binary actin-ADP-ribosylating toxin, binary toxin (CDT). CDT leads to the disruption of the actin cytoskeleton, leading to the formation of microtubule-based cell protrusions, allowing enhanced colonization of the gut epithelium by *C difficile*.[25] These CDT-induced protrusions are involved in vesicular transport. CDT reroutes Rab11-positive vesicles containing fibronectin, which is involved in bacterial adherence, leading to the increased adherence of *C difficile*, one of the first steps of colonization. Although it has been speculated that the binary toxin has an additive effect to damage already caused by the other 2 toxins, Kuehne and colleagues[26] created knock-out combinations of isogenic toxin mutants of R20291 and assessed their virulence in hamsters. An isogenic mutant ($A^-B^-C^+$) that produces only CDT was able to cause disease in a third of the hamsters tested, although symptoms vary from those typically associated with CDI. Signs of wet tail, hemorrhage, and inflammation in their small intestines were observed, suggesting an independent role of CDT in causing disease.

C difficile spores play an important role in disease pathogenesis. Spores can survive in the environment for long periods of time and are generally resistant to household cleaners and antimicrobials. Because of the importance of spores in the transmission of CDI, germination rates of hypervirulent *C difficile* BI/NAP1/027 have been studied in great detail. Initial studies comparing the germination efficiencies of *C difficile* BI/NAP1/027 and historic *C difficile* strain 630 suggested that hypervirulent strains may have higher germination efficiencies. Most recent studies looking at a greater number of strains have displayed intraclade and interclade differences in germination efficiencies.[27,28]

The genome of hypervirulent *C difficile* BI/NAP1/027 has been shown to contain a large number of mobile genetic elements that code for a variety of antibiotic-resistant genes. At the turn of the century, the most commonly prescribed antibiotic was fluoroquinolone, and the rapid spread of hypervirulent *C difficile* BI/NAP1/027 could also be due to the highly fluoroquinolone-resistant phenotype of these strains because of point mutations on the DNA gyrase genes.[29]

Although the spread of hypervirulent *C difficile* BI/NAP1/027 is continuing in certain geographic areas while decreasing in others, it is likely that in future outbreaks new epidemic strains will emerge with very different profiles. In Europe, for example, *C difficile* ribotype 078 is the most common circulating ribotype in community-acquired CDI cases, whereas *C difficile* ribotype 027 is increasingly associated with severe cases of CDI.[30]

The Importance of Vaccines Against Clostridium difficile Infection

Multiple studies using computer simulation and databases demonstrate that CDI is a costly disease, with an added expense of $1 to 3 billion annually in the United States. This added economic burden is borne by hospitals, by patients and their families, and by society.[31] Mild cases of CDI can lead to added costs and lengthened hospital stays, whereas severe cases with complications such as toxic megacolon and sepsis can lead to expensive surgical procedures, intensive care unit stays, and even death. A recent study looked at the economic burden of CDI on cardiac surgical patients alone using the Nationwide Inpatient Sample database and reported that, in cardiac surgery alone, CDI adds an incremental cost of $212 million per year.[32] The aging US population combined with limited health care dollars requires the development of novel approaches to stop this CDI epidemic.

Although the spread of *C difficile* may be reduced and prevented by strict adherence to hand hygiene and other contact precautions, such as patient isolation, stringent use of antimicrobials, and rigorous environmental cleaning, such control practices are costly and even bundle approaches have not yet yielded the desired results. Prophylactic and therapeutic vaccines against *C difficile* may be the best way to end the expansion and spread of this nosocomial disease. Mathematical studies of CDI suggest the possible benefits of herd immunity in controlling disease transmission.[33] Vaccination to prevent CDI appears to be cost-effective based on computer-simulation models in a variety of circumstances with varying CDI risks, vaccine costs, and vaccine efficacies.[33] An effective *C difficile* vaccine could be considered for both prophylactic and therapeutic applications in several target populations, for example, patients likely to be admitted to the hospital and receive antibiotics, including those presenting for emergency room visits, and before elective or urgent surgical procedures. Similarly, at-risk patients in long-term care facilities such as nursing homes and hospices could be vaccinated on admission. Patients who have had one episode of CDI are at a high risk of recurrent CDI and could be targeted for vaccination to prevent recurrence.

IMPORTANCE OF HOST IMMUNE RESPONSES IN *CLOSTRIDIUM DIFFICILE* INFECTION

The host immune response to CDI is an important predictor of disease outcome, with outcomes ranging from asymptomatic intestinal colonization to diarrhea, colitis, pseudomembranous colitis, and, in severe cases, sepsis and death. The mechanisms of innate immune responses against C difficile and its toxins remain unclear. It is also unclear whether these responses are protective, deleterious, or a combination of these. On the other hand, the role of adaptive immune responses against TcdA and TcdB has been studied in greater detail and are known to be capable of positively influencing disease outcomes (**Table 1**).

Innate Immune Responses to Clostridium difficile Infection

Innate immune responses to C difficile have been studied in animal models of CDI, ex vivo studies using human cell lines and mucosal explants, and a limited number of studies in CDI patients.[34] The innate defense mechanisms against CDI include the host's normal microbiota and the mucosal immune system, which includes intestinal epithelial cells. The human gut contains a normal microbiota consisting of diverse bacterial species that maintain a metabolic equilibrium in the gut. Production of cationic antimicrobial peptides (CAMPs), such as polymixin or nisin, by the gut microbiota helps maintain colonization resistance, which allows the resident microbiota to out-compete pathogens for niches and nutrients.[35] Specifically for C difficile, gut microbiota regulate the production of sodium taurocholate, a bile salt analogue needed for the germination of C difficile spores to its disease-causing vegetative form, thereby controlling the lifecycle of C difficile.[36] Following antibiotic administration, the diversity of the gut microflora is reduced, allowing a pathogenic bacterium like C difficile to out-compete the resident gut microbiota, germinate to substantial levels, and produce disease-causing toxins.

Toxin production during CDI leads to an inflammatory response that includes the production of pro-inflammatory cytokines and chemokines, including interleukin (IL)-8, IL-12, IL-18, interferon γ (IFN-γ), IL-1β, tumor necrosis factor (TNF)-α, and macrophage inflammatory protein 1α (MIP-1α), which may be responsible for damage to gut epithelial cells. These toxins also lead to the activation of toll-like receptor 4 (TLR-4), NOD1, and the IL-1β/inflammasome.[37] Neutrophil activation, aided by mast cell degranulation, can lead to extensive host cell damage. Activation of innate immune sensors, followed by the release of cytokines and chemokines, are followed by local neutrophilic infiltration, a hallmark of CDI. Most studies show that activation of a pro-inflammatory innate immune response leads to increased damage to the gut; however, a few studies point to the fact that a lack of neutrophil recruitment may lead to poor control of C difficile burden, and a worsening of CDI.

Other C difficile surface proteins like flagellin activate TLR-5.[38] The role of flagellin in the activation of TLR-5 may lead to protection against CDI-induced damage. Therefore, it is still unknown whether innate immune responses are, as a whole, beneficial or harmful to the human host.

Natural Adaptive Immune Responses to Clostridium difficile Infection

Clinical research study findings indicate that host immune responses play an important role in determining the manifestations and outcomes of CDI.[39] Although fewer than 5% of adults and older children are colonized, antibodies against C difficile are

Table 1
Immune responses to *Clostridium difficile*

Adaptive Immunity	Role in CID
Antitoxin antibodies	Anti-TcdA and Anti-TcdB antibodies
	Antitoxin antibodies are present in most adults and older children through transient exposure to *C difficile*
Antibodies against nontoxin antigens	Antibodies against surface proteins like flagella and protease Cwp84
	Antibodies against adhesion molecules

Innate Immunity	Role in CID
Host's intestinal microbiota	Competitive inhibition/exclusion for niche and nutrients
	Production of CAMPs to help maintain colonization resistance
	Regulation of the production of sodium taurocholate, which is needed for *C difficile* spore germination
(Intestinal) mucosal immune system	Production of cytokines and chemokines such as IL-8, IL-1, IL-18, IFN-γ, IL-1β, TNF-α, and MIP-1α
	Activation of TRL-4, NOD1, and the IL-1β/inflammasome
	Activation of TRL-5 by flagellin
	Neutrophil activation and mast cell degranulation

present in most adults and older children, presumably through transient exposure to *C difficile* toxins either during infancy or from the environment in adulthood. *C difficile* spores are present ubiquitously in the soil, in meat and poultry, and in domestic and wild animals. Multiple studies suggest that, following exposure, immune responses to *C difficile* and its toxins influence the development and clinical course of CDI.[40–43]

Seminal work looking at serum and fecal antibody responses to *C difficile* TcdA, TcdB, and nontoxin antigens over time in a prospective study of 271 hospitalized patients receiving antibiotics reported that, at the time of colonization, asymptomatic carriers of *C difficile* had significantly higher serum immunoglobulin G (IgG) antibody levels to TcdA compared with colonized patients who later developed CDI.[39] In addition, asymptomatic carriers also showed greater immune responses to TcdB and nontoxin antigens, although these differences were not as significant, possibly because of small sample sizes.[39,44] Antitoxin antibody levels were shown to be independent of age, comorbidity, or severity of underlying disease; however, the effect of higher serum IgG anti-TcdA levels in protecting against CDI was less marked in very ill patients. Conversely, recent studies have reported similar levels of serum IgG and IgM antibody levels against crude and purified TcdA in colonized patients with and without CDI, and matched controls.[45]

The role of mucosal immune responses against CDI and the toxins is not well-defined in patients, although a few studies suggest that high mucosal anti-TcdA IgA antibody concentrations as well as the presence of antitoxin antibodies in stool are associated with protection against severe CDI. In a mouse model of CDI, C57BL/6 mice $pIgR^{-/-}$ mice, lacking the receptor to transcytose polymeric antibodies, were also protected from CDI, suggesting that polymeric mucosal antitoxin antibodies are not essential for protection (ie, protection against CDI can be mediated through simple exudation of serum antitoxin IgG across the inflamed intestinal epithelium).[46] This theory is in keeping with the associations between serum IgG antitoxin concentrations and clinical outcomes of CDI as discussed earlier. It is also in keeping with the demonstrated clinical efficacy of serum IgG antitoxin in protecting against recurrent CDI in humans as discussed later.

Adaptive Immune Responses in Recurrent Clostridium difficile Infection

Acquired immunity during an initial episode of CDI results in a serum antitoxin immunoglobulin response that can protect against recurrent CDI, which is a major clinical problem afflicting more than 25% of CDI patients.[44] In patients with CDI, serum IgM levels against TcdA, TcdB, and nontoxin antigens were significantly higher in patients who had a single episode of diarrhea compared with patients who later developed recurrent CDI, when measured as early as day 3 (for IgM) following symptomatic disease.[44] Recurrent CDI also correlates well with a failure to mount effective neutralizing serum anti-toxin IgG by day 12 of initial infection.[44] Therefore, CDI patients who can mount an immune response early in the course of their illness are less likely to go on to develop recurrent CDI. In one small study, patients lacking IgG_2 and IgG_3 subclass anti-TcdA IgG antibodies were found to be at a higher risk for recurrent CDI.[47]

Antibody responses to TcdA initially demonstrated the strongest association with protection from disease in both animal models and human cohort studies.[44,48] However, multiple lines of evidence indicate that an effective vaccine will likely need to neutralize both toxins A and B to be most effective in protecting against symptomatic disease.[5,49,50] Furthermore, to prevent colonization and disease transmission, it is highly likely that nontoxin antigens will also need to be targeted.[39]

Preliminary in vivo experiments using the targeted ClosTron gene knock-out system for the genus *Clostridium* indicates a redundancy of function within the surface-associated proteins that mediate adherence.[51] Nevertheless, recent clinical studies in patients with CDI suggest that antibody levels against surface proteins such as flagella and protease Cwp84 are significantly higher in a group of protected patients as compared with a CDI patient group.[52] This finding suggests that these proteins may be able to induce an immune response that could play a role in defense against colonization, albeit that the role of such antibodies in interrupting the pathogenesis of CDI is unknown.

The virulence of C difficile is due to a complex multifactorial interplay between several known virulence factors, such as the toxins and the adhesion molecules. TcdA and TcdB are essential for symptomatic disease, whereas additional virulence factors, such as flagellar proteins, have been implicated in motility and biofilm formation and may also influence toxin production. Taken together, these factors suggest that development of a commercially viable C difficile vaccine suitable for the broadest range of indications would likely target a single factor or multiple factors needed for colonization, persistence, and toxin production; this may present a significant advantage over several vaccines currently in development that solely target toxin neutralization. Whatever the approach, vaccination represents a very valuable strategy to prevent and control CDI.

PASSIVE IMMUNOTHERAPY AGAINST CLOSTRIDIUM DIFFICILE INFECTION

Given the importance of the humoral response against toxins, and possibly against nontoxin determinants of CDI, passive immunization of a susceptible host with monoclonal antibodies could provide both a preventive and a therapeutic passive immunization strategy. Recent breakthrough developments in monoclonal antibody research allow for diverse ways of isolating monoclonal antibodies other than the historical method of purifying antibodies from hybridomas. Novel methods of isolating monoclonal antibodies from single B cells, from either hyperimmunized mice or infected patients, isolation of recombinant single domain antibody fragments from immune llama phage display libraries, isolation of antisera from hyperimmunized sheep, horses, and chicken have all aided in the identification of monoclonal antibodies against C difficile, with toxins being the most commonly used target.[53] Passive immunization with monoclonal antibodies may be used as prophylaxis in high-risk patients unable to mount an effective immune response at a critical time in their illness, as therapy in patients with fulminant or refractory CDI or to reduce the rate of recurrence in patients who are likely to have a reduced response to active immunization.

Passive Immunization Against Clostridium difficile Infection in Animals

Passive immunization via oral or parenteral administration of antitoxin antibody formulations has been shown to protect antibiotic-treated mice and hamsters from lethal challenge with C difficile spores (**Table 2**). Formulations of colostrum from cows immunized with C difficile toxoids were shown to protect hamsters from death caused by CDI.[54] Avian immunoglobulins in the form of egg IgY antibodies against recombinant peptides spanning the TcdA and TcdB when given orogastrically to hamsters provided complete protection from CDI and death.[55] Ovine hyperimmune serum against different regions of the RBDs of the toxins has helped narrow down the essential regions needed for a toxin-neutralizing immune response to protect against disease and death.[56] Fully human monoclonal antibodies against the RBD of TcdA and TcdB have been developed by many groups and a combination of these parenterally given monoclonal antibodies were shown to protect antibiotic-treated mice or hamsters from C difficile challenge.[49,57,58]

Table 2

Immunization against toxins and cell-surface proteins in clinical and animal trials

Targets	Immunization	Clinical Trials	Animal Trials
Toxins	Passive	1. IVIG has shown protective efficacy in patients from primary and recurrent CDI. 2. Human monoclonal antibodies CDA-1 and CDB-2 have been tested in a phase I open-label dose escalation study. They were also tested in 200 patients that were recovering from an initial episode of CDI in a phase II multicenter, randomized, double-blind, placebo-controlled trial. The result was a 72% relative reduction in recurrence rates as compared with a placebo.	1. Formulations of colostrum from cows immunized with *C difficile* toxins were shown to protect hamsters from CDI and death. 2. Equine hyperimmune serum was able to protect against a *C difficile* spore challenge in a murine model of CDI. 3. Avian immunoglobulins in the form of egg IgY antibodies given to hamsters provided complete protection from CDI and death. 4. Human monoclonal antibodies against the RBD of TcdA and TcdB were shown to protect antibiotic-treated mice or hamsters from a *C difficile* challenge.
	Active	1. The vaccine, licensed by Sanofi Pasteur, containing formalin-inactivated purified toxins A and B adjuvanted with alum has been tested in 6 phase I trials in more than 200 volunteers and was found to be safe and well tolerated. 2. The vaccine developed by Pfizer, containing toxoids A and B, is currently being tested in a phase I, placebo-controlled, randomized, observer-blinded study. 3. Intercell has initiated a phase I, open-labeled dose-escalation study of its recombinant protein in healthy adults to test the safety of a recombinant protein-based parenteral vaccine consisting of truncated TcdA and TcdB.	1. Recombinantly produced domains of the toxins have been shown to be immunogenic, capable of inducing neutralizing antibodies, and protective against bacterial challenge in murine and hamster model of CDI. 2. Merck Research Laboratories are developing a 4-component vaccine that targets TcdA, TcdB as well as the 2 components of the binary toxin, CdtA and CdtB. This vaccine leads to full protection against lethal challenge with the *C difficile* BI/NAP1/r027 strain in hamsters.
Cell-surface proteins	Active		1. Immunization with SLPs with various adjuvants provided only partial protection against a *C difficile* challenge in hamsters. 2. The immunogenicity of conjugate vaccines of PSII fused with various carrier proteins, such as fragments of TcdA and TcdB, has been studied in mice and hamsters and are found to be immunogenic. 3. Using *B subtilis* spores to express BclA1 on CotB demonstrated 40% protection in hamsters following oral immunization.

Passive Immunization Against Clostridium difficile Infection in Humans

Few clinical studies in humans have looked at the efficacy of using normal pooled immunoglobulin preparations that contain toxin-neutralizing activity. In early clinical studies, the intravenous immunoglobulin G fraction (IVIG) has been reported to be effective in a small number of patients suffering from a severe or recurrent CDI.[59,60] Different doses, varying frequencies of administration, given with or without antibiotics, have since produced varying results.[61] The general consensus is that IVIG may ameliorate patient disease when CDI is confined to the colon; however, in patients who have systemic symptoms such as multiorgan dysfunction, IVIG is found to less beneficial. The lack of large-scale, randomized and controlled studies has prevented a thorough study of the benefits of IVIG in severe or recurrent CDI.

Fully human monoclonal antibodies have been developed and tested in humans as a treatment of CDI. Medarex, Inc and Massachusetts Biological Laboratories have developed human monoclonal antibodies, CDA-1 and CDB-1, to the RBDs of TcdA and TcdB, respectively.[62,63] Following the demonstration of their efficacy in hamsters, a phase I open-label dose escalation study in 30 healthy volunteers demonstrated that these antibodies, given as an intravenous infusion of CDA-1, are well-tolerated, with no serious adverse events.[64] Interestingly, in a subsequent small phase 2 study, the infusion of CDA-1 alone did not appear to be highly effective. These humanized monoclonal antibodies, given as an adjunct to standard antimicrobial therapy, were then tested in 200 patients recovering from an initial episode of CDI in a phase 2 multicenter, randomized, double-blind, placebo-controlled trial for the prevention of CDI recurrence.[49,62,63] The combination antibody treatment was safe and well tolerated and had circulating half-lives of up to 26 days. Treatment was associated with a 72% relative reduction in recurrence rates compared with placebo. This antibody therapy did not significantly reduce the severity of the diarrheal illness, the duration of hospitalization, or the time to resolution of the diarrhea.[63] Studies are now underway to determine whether these monoclonal antibodies can afford protection against recurrent CDI or reduce disease duration or severity. Given the high costs of monoclonal antibody therapies, it is unlikely that these antibodies will be developed as primary prophylaxis unless extremely high-risk groups can be identified.

These studies support the theory that the correlate of protection against CDI is the presence of high serum antitoxin IgG. The mechanism by which serum antitoxin IgG is able to protect against toxin-mediated damage in the mucosa of the colon is still unclear. It is certainly possible that serum antitoxin IgG is exuded into the gut lumen because of the increased permeability of the intestinal epithelial cell layer caused by TcdA and TcdB. FcRN receptors present in the epithelial cells of the gut are able to transport IgG across the intestinal epithelium; however, recent studies in mice indicate that FcRN is not required for IgG antitoxin-mediated protection (Zhang Z, Chen X, Hernandez L, et al, unpublished observations, 2014).[65] Regardless of the mechanisms and sites whereby IgG antitoxins neutralize TcdA and TcdB, the clinical studies and human trial discussed earlier confirm the importance of serum antitoxin antibodies in protecting against CDI; this consolidates the importance of pursuing both passive and active immunization regimens to protect against CDI.

ACTIVE VACCINATION AGAINST CLOSTRIDIUM DIFFICILE INFECTION

The ability to stimulate toxin-neutralizing responses is likely to be a key property of a protective CDI vaccine and, to date, the best correlate of vaccine efficacy is the development of serum neutralizing antibodies against both toxins.[39,44,62,63,66–71] Over the past decade, a variety of vaccines targeting the toxins have been tested in animals and a few have progressed to human clinical trials, although none are US Food and Drug Administration–approved for human use (see **Table 2**).

Active Vaccination Against Clostridium difficile Infection Targeting the Toxins

The first candidate vaccine against *C difficile* that has been tested in humans is a toxoid-based vaccine containing formalin-inactivated purified TcdA and TcdB adjuvanted with alum and administered as 3 parenteral doses. This vaccine, under development by Sanofi Pasteur, has been tested in 6 phase 1 trials in more than 200 volunteers.[72] In healthy volunteers, intramuscular administration of this vaccine was found to be safe and well-tolerated, with no vaccine-related serious adverse events reported. One study found that seroconversion to TcdB was less frequent than to TcdA.[73] Seroconversion was less common in elderly subjects ($\geq$65 years), who are the expected target population, as compared with younger adults (18–55 years). The requirement for 3 administrations of this vaccine to achieve protective serum antitoxin antibody levels may limit its use to longer-term prevention rather than prevention in those at imminent risk for CDI.[74,75] Several phase II studies of the vaccine have been performed. The first was designed to study the effect of the vaccine on patients with multiple recurrences of CDI; vaccination was able to successfully treat a small number of such patients (3 patients).[71] A second study was designed to compare the incidence of recurrent CDI in the 9-week period after the third dose of the vaccine in subjects with a first episode of CDI treated with standard-of-care antibiotics and either vaccine or placebo. The study was halted due to slow enrollment, and efficacy data have not been released as of yet. A phase III study is now recruiting healthy adults aged 50 to 85 years at risk for CDI and has an expected completion date in 2015. Stated outcome measures include vaccine safety, tolerability, and immunogenicity.

Parenterally delivered toxoid-based vaccines are also being developed by Pfizer. To avoid residual toxicity issues with formalin inactivation, Pfizer's toxoid-based vaccine is first rendered 10,000-fold less toxic by the introduction of targeted mutations in the N-terminal glucosyltransferase cytotoxicity domains. This mutation is followed by formalin treatment to remove the residual toxicity as assayed by in vitro cell-based toxicity assays.[76] Phase 1 studies in healthy adult volunteers have examined an alum-adjuvanted vaccine, containing toxoid A and B, administered in 3 parenteral doses, to evaluate safety and immunogenicity.[77]

Holotoxins are difficult to purify and produce, require formalin inactivation, tend to be unstable and to degrade over time, and contain some contaminating antigens. To circumvent these problems, recombinant toxin domains have been produced and shown to be immunogenic, capable of inducing neutralizing antibodies, and to provide protection against bacterial challenge in murine and hamster models of CDI.[38] Multiple laboratories and pharmaceutical companies are working on various domains of TcdA and TcdB to identify epitopes that have potent and protective toxin neutralizing ability in vitro and in vivo. A fusion protein containing the RBDs of TcdA and TcdB has been produced and shown to induce protective immunity against *C difficile* toxins in hamsters.[78] Valneva (formerly Intercell) has completed a phase 1, open-label study of this recombinant protein, with or without aluminum hydroxide as an adjuvant; good safety, tolerability, and immunogenicity profiles were seen in both healthy adults and healthy at-risk volunteers aged 65 years and older.[79]

Given the potential importance of mucosal immunity in CDI, delivery of a vaccine by a mucosal route using a mucosal adjuvant may be advantageous. *Bacillus subtilis* spores have been used as a vaccine delivery agent because antigens can be displayed on the spore surface. The modified spores are inactivated and then used for mucosal immunization, by either oral, sublingual, or nasal routes. *Bacillus* spores carry a natural adjuvant property that leads to a balanced Th1 and Th2 response.[80] CDVAX is a novel *B subtilis* vaccine expressing a fragment of TcdA fused to CotB and CotC surface proteins of *B subtilis*. The vaccine is able to induce serum and fecal antibodies that neutralize TcdB and is protective in hamsters following oral administration of *B subtilis* PP108 (CotB-A26-39 CotC-A2639).[81] This vaccine is now in early stages of clinical development.

In addition to TcdA and TcdB, hypervirulent strains of *C difficile* BI/NAP1/027 strains express the binary toxin CDT. Therefore, it may be valuable to target CDT as an added component of a *C difficile* vaccine. Merck Research Laboratories are developing a multivalent vaccine that targets TcdA, TcdB as well as the 2 components of the CDT, CdtA and CdtB.[82,83] Mutations in the active enzymatic sites of TcdA, TcdB, and CDT lead to reduced toxicity in animal models of CDI. This 4-component vaccine leads to full protection against lethal challenge with epidemic *C difficile* BI/NAP1/r027 strain in hamsters and is also in the early stages of clinical development.

Active Vaccination Against Clostridium difficile Infection Targeting Surface Proteins

Colonization of the host by *C difficile* is an important step in the disease pathogenesis of CDI. Although a strong immune response against TcdA and TcdB may prevent the development of disease, it does not prevent colonization of the host by the bacterium. Various adherence factors, such as S-layer protein (SLPs), flagellar proteins, FliC and FliD, protease Cwp84, the Fbp68 fibronectin binding protein, and the GroEL heat-shock protein, have been studied as potential vaccine candidates in animals. However, preliminary experiments using knock-out strains in animal models suggest a redundancy of function within the surface-associated proteins that are associated with adherence and colonization.[51,84]

C difficile is surrounded by a paracrystalline S-layer that consists of a high-molecular-weight SLP and a low-molecular-weight SLP.[85] SLPs can activate innate and adaptive immunity via TLR4.[86] Although SLPs are able to bind gastrointestinal tissues, active immunization with SLPs with various adjuvants provided only partial protection against *C difficile* challenge in hamsters.[87] In a human clinical study, however, patients with recurrent CDI had significantly lower IgM-anti-SLP levels than patients with a single episode, suggesting that anti-SLP immune responses might be protective.

C difficile flagellar proteins play myriad roles in disease pathogenesis from adherence, toxin production, and biofilm formation. These roles are also strain-specific. Given the importance of flagella in the virulence of *C difficile*, active immunization of a susceptible host using *C difficile* flagellar components in addition to TcdA and TcdB could provide both a preventive and a therapeutic vaccine strategy, by reducing or preventing bacterial colonization as well as preventing toxin-induced disease. *C difficile* flagellum is made up of 2 components, the 39-kDa FliC (flagellin) and the 56-kDa flagellar cap protein FliD.[88,89] Several studies have reported that the flagella proteins are highly immunogenic, and during the course of natural infection, antiflagella immune responses may play a role in protection against colonization.[52,90] These flagellar proteins may also be developed as targets for passive immunotherapy in the form of monoclonal antibodies.

The vegetative form of *C difficile* cells contains 3 highly complex cell-surface polysaccharides (PSI, PSII, and PSIII).[91] PSII is abundantly expressed by all *C difficile* ribotypes, including the hypervirulent *C difficile* BI/NAP1/r027 strains.[92] Conjugate vaccines of PSII fused with various carrier proteins, such as fragments of TcdA and TcdB, have been found to be immunogenic in animals. Further studies are underway to elucidate the role of anti-PSII adaptive immune responses against *C difficile* colonization.[93]

C difficile spores play an important role in disease pathogenesis. Germination of spores into vegetative cells is a critical step in the lifecycle of *C difficile*, and interrupting this event can prevent subsequent colonization, toxin production, CDI, and disease transmission. Spore proteins present on the outer layer of spores, the exosporium, may be essential for the initiation and persistence of CDI. Pizarro-Guajardo and colleagues[94] reported that 3 *C difficile* collagenlike exosporium proteins (BclA1, BclA2, and BclA3) are expressed during sporulation and localize to the spore; however, the role of *C difficile* BclA proteins in spore-host interactions remains unclear. BclA1, an ortholog in *Bacillus anthracis* spores that has been shown to protect immunized mice from *B anthracis* spore colonization, is a potential vaccine candidate for CDI. Using *B subtilis* spores to express BclA1 on CotB afforded 40% protection in hamsters following oral immunization. The addition of TcdA and/or TcdB as vaccine components may allow for targeting of both the spore and the toxins to further improve the level of protection. *C difficile* spore proteins, such as BclA1, CotB, CdeC, and others, may also be developed as potential targets for passive immunotherapy in the form of monoclonal antibodies.[95]

Glycoproteins present on both spores as well as the vegetative cells are attractive targets for vaccine development. One such example is lipoteichoic acid (LTA), which is conserved across most *C difficile* strains.[96] Immunization of mice and hamsters with LTA conjugated to a carrier protein with a maleimide-thiol linker was immunogenic and was able to afford partial protection against lethal bacterial challenge.

SUMMARY

In the last decade, disease caused by *C difficile* has increased and spread across the globe at an alarming rate. This new epidemic of CDI with increases in both morbidity and mortality has been associated with the emergence of highly virulent *C difficile* strains, most notably BI/NAP1/027. Although the pathogenesis of CDI is closely linked to toxins A and B, several other factors, such as SLPs and flagellar proteins, have been shown to play an important role in disease pathogenesis. *C difficile* spores can survive in the environment for long periods of time and are resistant to most household cleaners and antimicrobial agents, making these a significant factor in the transmission of CDI. Despite the current approaches to prevention and treatment of CDI, the incidence, morbidity, mortality, and cost of the infection continue to increase at an alarming pace. Given the importance of the humoral response against CDI, novel approaches toward prophylactic and therapeutic vaccines, involving either active or passive vaccination, provide an attractive alternative approach to stem the spread of CDI.

REFERENCES

1. Bartlett JG, Moon N, Chang TW, et al. Role of Clostridium difficile in antibiotic-associated pseudomembranous colitis. Gastroenterology 1978;75:778–82.
2. Kelly CP. Current strategies for management of initial Clostridium difficile infection. J Hosp Med 2012;7(Suppl 3):S5–10.
3. Bassis CM, Theriot CM, Young VB. Alteration of the murine gastrointestinal microbiota by tigecycline leads to increased susceptibility to Clostridium difficile infection. Antimicrob Agents Chemother 2014;58:2767–74.
4. Theriot CM, Koenigsknecht MJ, Carlson PE Jr, et al. Antibiotic-induced shifts in the mouse gut microbiome and metabolome increase susceptibility to Clostridium difficile infection. Nat Commun 2014;5:3114.
5. Kuehne SA, Cartman ST, Heap JT, et al. The role of toxin A and toxin B in Clostridium difficile infection. Nature 2010;467:711–3.

6. Hundsberger T, Braun V, Weidmann M, et al. Transcription analysis of the genes tcdA-E of the pathogenicity locus of Clostridium difficile. Eur J Biochem 1997; 244:735–42.

7. Voth DE, Ballard JD. Clostridium difficile toxins: mechanism of action and role in disease. Clin Microbiol Rev 2005;18:247–63.

8. Jank T, Giesemann T, Aktories K. Rho-glucosylating Clostridium difficile toxins A and B: new insights into structure and function. Glycobiology 2007;17:15R–22R.

9. Jank T, Aktories K. Structure and mode of action of clostridial glucosylating toxins: the ABCD model. Trends Microbiol 2008;16:222–9.

10. Ho JG, Greco A, Rupnik M, et al. Crystal structure of receptor-binding C-terminal repeats from Clostridium difficile toxin A. Proc Natl Acad Sci U S A 2005;102: 18373–8.

11. Greco A, Ho JG, Lin SJ, et al. Carbohydrate recognition by Clostridium difficile toxin A. Nat Struct Mol Biol 2006;13:460–1.

12. Jank T, Giesemann T, Aktories K. Clostridium difficile glucosyltransferase toxin B-essential amino acids for substrate binding. J Biol Chem 2007;282:35222–31.

13. Lyerly DM, Lockwood DE, Richardson SH, et al. Biological-activities of toxin-a and toxin-B of Clostridium-difficile. Infect Immun 1982;35:1147–50.

14. Johnson S, Kent SA, O'Leary KJ, et al. Fatal pseudomembranous colitis associated with a variant clostridium difficile strain not detected by toxin A immunoassay. Ann Intern Med 2001;135:434–8.

15. Drudy D, Fanning S, Kyne L. Toxin A-negative, toxin B-positive Clostridium difficile. Int J Infect Dis 2007;11:5–10.

16. Kasendra M, Barrile R, Leuzzi R, et al. Clostridium difficile toxins facilitate bacterial colonization by modulating the fence and gate function of colonic epithelium. J Infect Dis 2013;209:1095–104.

17. McDonald LC, Owings M, Jernigan DB. Clostridium difficile infection in patients discharged from US short-stay hospitals, 1996-2003. Emerg Infect Dis 2006;12: 409–15.

18. Bartlett JG, Perl TM. The new Clostridium difficile–what does it mean? N Engl J Med 2005;353:2503–5.

19. He M, Miyajima F, Roberts P, et al. Emergence and global spread of epidemic healthcare-associated Clostridium difficile. Nat Genet 2013;45:109–13.

20. Miller BA, Chen LF, Sexton DJ, et al. Comparison of the burdens of hospital-onset, healthcare facility-associated Clostridium difficile Infection and of healthcare-associated infection due to methicillin-resistant Staphylococcus aureus in community hospitals. Infect Control Hosp Epidemiol 2011;32:387–90.

21. Eyre DW, Cule ML, Wilson DJ, et al. Diverse sources of C. difficile infection identified on whole-genome sequencing. N Engl J Med 2013;369:1195–205.

22. Khanna S, Pardi DS, Aronson SL, et al. The epidemiology of community-acquired Clostridium difficile infection: a population-based study. Am J Gastroenterol 2012;107:89–95.

23. Dupuy B, Govind R, Antunes A, et al. Clostridium difficile toxin synthesis is negatively regulated by TcdC. J Med Microbiol 2008;57:685–9.

24. Lanis JM, Barua S, Ballard JD. Variations in TcdB activity and the hypervirulence of emerging strains of Clostridium difficile. PLoS Pathog 2010;6:e1001061.

25. Schwan C, Stecher B, Tzivelekidis T, et al. Clostridium difficile toxin CDT induces formation of microtubule-based protrusions and increases adherence of bacteria. PLoS Pathog 2009;5:e1000626.

26. Kuehne SA, Collery MM, Kelly ML, et al. Importance of toxin A, toxin B, and CDT in virulence of an epidemic Clostridium difficile strain. J Infect Dis 2014;209:83–6.

27. Merrigan M, Venugopal A, Mallozzi M, et al. Human hypervirulent Clostridium difficile strains exhibit increased sporulation as well as robust toxin production. J Bacteriol 2010;192:4904–11.

28. Heeg D, Burns DA, Cartman ST, et al. Spores of Clostridium difficile clinical isolates display a diverse germination response to bile salts. PLoS One 2012;7: e32381.

29. Brouwer MS, Warburton PJ, Roberts AP, et al. Genetic organisation, mobility and predicted functions of genes on integrated, mobile genetic elements in sequenced strains of Clostridium difficile. PLoS One 2011;6:e23014.

30. Jones AM, Kuijper EJ, Wilcox MH. Clostridium difficile: a European perspective. J Infect 2013;66:115–28.

31. McGlone SM, Bailey RR, Zimmer SM, et al. The economic burden of Clostridium difficile. Clin Microbiol Infect 2012;18:282–9.

32. Flagg A, Koch CG, Schiltz N, et al. Analysis of Clostridium difficilse infections after cardiac surgery: epidemiologic and economic implications from national data. J Thorac Cardiovasc Surg 2014;148:2404–9.

33. Lee BY, Popovich MJ, Tian Y, et al. The potential value of Clostridium difficile vaccine: an economic computer simulation model. Vaccine 2010;28:5245–53.

34. Kelly CP, Kyne L. The host immune response to Clostridium difficile. J Med Microbiol 2011;60:1070–9.

35. Lawley TD, Walker AW. Intestinal colonization resistance. Immunology 2013;138: 1–11.

36. Britton RA, Young VB. Role of the intestinal microbiota in resistance to colonization by Clostridium difficile. Gastroenterology 2014;146:1547–53.

37. Madan R, Petri WA. Immune responses to Clostridium difficile infection. Trends Mol Med 2012;18:658–66.

38. Ghose C, Verhagen JM, Chen X, et al. Toll-like receptor 5-dependent immunogenicity and protective efficacy of a recombinant fusion protein vaccine containing the nontoxic domains of clostridium difficile toxins A and B and Salmonella enterica serovar typhimurium flagellin in a mouse model of Clostridium difficile disease. Infect Immun 2013;81:2190–6.

39. Kyne L, Warny M, Qamar A, et al. Asymptomatic carriage of Clostridium difficile and serum levels of IgG antibody against toxin A. N Engl J Med 2000;342:390–7.

40. Aronsson B, Granstrom M, Mollby R, et al. Serum antibody response to Clostridium difficile toxins in patients with Clostridium difficile diarrhoea. Infection 1985;13:97–101.

41. Mulligan ME, Miller SD, McFarland LV, et al. Elevated levels of serum immunoglobulins in asymptomatic carriers of Clostridium difficile. Clin Infect Dis 1993; 16(Suppl 4):S239–44.

42. Johnson S, Gerding DN, Janoff EN. Systemic and mucosal antibody responses to toxin A in patients infected with Clostridium difficile. J Infect Dis 1992;166: 1287–94.

43. Warny M, Vaerman JP, Avesani V, et al. Human antibody response to Clostridium difficile toxin A in relation to clinical course of infection. Infect Immun 1994;62: 384–9.

44. Kyne L, Warny M, Qamar A, et al. Association between antibody response to toxin A and protection against recurrent Clostridium difficile diarrhoea. Lancet 2001; 357:189–93.

45. Sanchez-Hurtado K, Corretge M, Mutlu E, et al. Systemic antibody response to Clostridium difficile in colonized patients with and without symptoms and matched controls. J Med Microbiol 2008;57:717–24.

46. Johnston PF, Gerding DN, Knight KL. Protection from Clostridium difficile infection in CD4 T Cell- and polymeric immunoglobulin receptor-deficient mice. Infect Immun 2014;82:522–31.

47. Katchar K, Taylor CP, Tummala S, et al. Association between IgG2 and IgG3 subclass responses to toxin A and recurrent Clostridium difficile-associated disease. Clin Gastroenterol Hepatol 2007;5:707–13.

48. Sambol SP, Tang JK, Merrigan MM, et al. Infection of hamsters with epidemiologically important strains of Clostridium difficile. J Infect Dis 2001;183:1760–6.

49. Babcock GJ, Broering TJ, Hernandez HJ, et al. Human monoclonal antibodies directed against toxins A and B prevent Clostridium difficile-induced mortality in hamsters. Infect Immun 2006;74:6339–47.

50. Loo VG, Bourgault AM, Poirier L, et al. Host and pathogen factors for Clostridium difficile infection and colonization. N Engl J Med 2011;365:1693–703.

51. Heap JT, Pennington OJ, Cartman ST, et al. The ClosTron: a universal gene knockout system for the genus Clostridium. J Microbiol Methods 2007;70:452–64.

52. Pechine S, Gleizes A, Janoir C, et al. Immunological properties of surface proteins of Clostridium difficile. J Med Microbiol 2005;54:193–6.

53. Gerding DN. Clostridium difficile infection prevention: biotherapeutics, immunologics, and vaccines. Discov Med 2012;13:75–83.

54. Lyerly DM, Bostwick EF, Binion SB, et al. Passive immunization of hamsters against disease caused by Clostridium difficile by use of bovine immunoglobulin G concentrate. Infect Immun 1991;59:2215–8.

55. Mulvey GL, Dingle TC, Fang L, et al. Therapeutic potential of egg yolk antibodies for treating Clostridium difficile infection. J Med Microbiol 2011;60:1181–7.

56. Roberts A, McGlashan J, Al-Abdulla I, et al. Development and evaluation of an ovine antibody-based platform for treatment of Clostridium difficile infection. Infect Immun 2012;80:875–82.

57. Davies NL, Compson JE, Mackenzie B, et al. A mixture of functionally oligoclonal humanized monoclonal antibodies that neutralize Clostridium difficile TcdA and TcdB with high levels of in vitro potency shows in vivo protection in a hamster infection model. Clin Vaccine Immunol 2013;20:377–90.

58. Marozsan AJ, Ma D, Nagashima KA, et al. Protection against Clostridium difficile infection with broadly neutralizing antitoxin monoclonal antibodies. J Infect Dis 2012;206:706–13.

59. Leung DY, Kelly CP, Boguniewicz M, et al. Treatment with intravenously administered gamma globulin of chronic relapsing colitis induced by Clostridium difficile toxin. J Pediatr 1991;118:633–7.

60. Salcedo J, Keates S, Pothoulakis C, et al. Intravenous immunoglobulin therapy for severe Clostridium difficile colitis. Gut 1997;41:366–70.

61. Abougergi MS, Kwon JH. Intravenous immunoglobulin for the treatment of Clostridium difficile infection: a review. Dig Dis Sci 2011;56:19–26.

62. Leav BA, Blair B, Leney M, et al. Serum anti-toxin B antibody correlates with protection from recurrent Clostridium difficile infection (CDI). Vaccine 2010;28:965–9.

63. Lowy I, Molrine DC, Leav BA, et al. Treatment with monoclonal antibodies against Clostridium difficile toxins. N Engl J Med 2010;362:197–205.

64. Taylor CP, Tummala S, Molrine D, et al. Open-label, dose escalation phase I study in healthy volunteers to evaluate the safety and pharmacokinetics of a human monoclonal antibody to Clostridium difficile toxin A. Vaccine 2008;26:3404–9.

65. Yoshida M, Masuda A, Kuo TT, et al. IgG transport across mucosal barriers by neonatal Fc receptor for IgG and mucosal immunity. Springer Semin Immunopathol 2006;28:397–403.

66. Torres J, Jennische E, Lange S, et al. Clostridium-difficile toxin-a induces a specific antisecretory factor which protects against intestinal mucosal damage. Gut 1991;32:791–5.

67. Torres JF, Lyerly DM, Hill JE, et al. Evaluation of formalin-inactivated Clostridium difficile vaccines administered by parenteral and mucosal routes of immunization in hamsters. Infect Immun 1995;63:4619–27.

68. Giannasca PJ, Zhang ZX, Lei WD, et al. Serum antitoxin antibodies mediate systemic and mucosal protection from Clostridium difficile disease in hamsters. Infect Immun 1999;67:527–38.

69. Giannasca PJ, Warny M. Active and passive immunization against Clostridium difficile diarrhea and colitis. Vaccine 2004;22:848–56.

70. Kyne L, Kelly CP. Prospects for a vaccine for Clostridium difficile. BioDrugs 1998; 10:173–81.

71. Sougioultzis S, Kyne L, Drudy D, et al. Clostridium difficile toxoid vaccine in recurrent C. difficile-associated diarrhea. Gastroenterology 2005;128:764–70.

72. Foglia G, Shah S, Luxemburger C, et al. Clostridium difficile: development of a novel candidate vaccine. Vaccine 2012;30:4307–9.

73. Greenberg RN, Marbury TC, Foglia G, et al. Phase I dose finding studies of an adjuvanted Clostridium difficile toxoid vaccine. Vaccine 2012;30:2245–9.

74. Kotloff KL, Wasserman SS, Losonsky GA, et al. Safety and immunogenicity of increasing doses of a Clostridium difficile toxoid vaccine administered to healthy adults. Infect Immun 2001;69:988–95.

75. Aboudola S, Kotloff KL, Kyne L, et al. Clostridium difficile vaccine and serum immunoglobulin G antibody response to toxin A. Infect Immun 2003;71: 1608–10.

76. Donald RG, Flint M, Kalyan N, et al. A novel approach to generate a recombinant toxoid vaccine against Clostridium difficile. Microbiology 2013;159:1254–66.

77. Pfizer. A study to investigate a clostridium difficile vaccine in healthy adults aged 50 to 85 years, who will each receive 3 doses of vaccine. In: ClinicalTrials.gov [Internet]. Bethesda (MD): National Library of Medicine (US). 2013 [cited 2014 December12]. Available at http://clinicaltrials.gov/ct2/show/ NCT02052726.

78. Tian JH, Fuhrmann SR, Kluepfel-Stahl S, et al. A novel fusion protein containing the receptor binding domains of C. difficile toxin A and toxin B elicits protective immunity against lethal toxin and spore challenge in preclinical efficacy models. Vaccine 2012;30:4249–58.

79. Valneva Austria GmbH. An open-label study assessing safety, immunogenicity and dose response of IC84. In: ClinicalTrials.gov [Internet]. Bethesda (MD): National Library of Medicine (US). 2011 [cited 2014 December12]. Available at: http://clinicaltrials.gov/ct2/show/NCT01296386?term=NCT01296386&rank=1.

80. Huang JM, La Ragione RM, Nunez A, et al. Immunostimulatory activity of Bacillus spores. FEMS Immunol Med Microbiol 2008;53:195–203.

81. Permpoonpattana P, Hong HA, Phetcharaburanin J, et al. Immunization with Bacillus spores expressing toxin A peptide repeats protects against infection with Clostridium difficile strains producing toxins A and B. Infect Immun 2011;79: 2295–302.

82. Karczewski J, Zorman J, Wang S, et al. Development of a recombinant toxin fragment vaccine for Clostridium difficile infection. Vaccine 2014;32:2812–8.

83. Xie J, Horton M, Zorman J, et al. Development and optimization of a high-throughput assay to measure neutralizing antibodies against Clostridium difficile binary toxin. Clin Vaccine Immunol 2014;21:689–97.

84. Wright A, Wait R, Begum S, et al. Proteomic analysis of cell surface proteins from Clostridium difficile. Proteomics 2005;5:2443–52.
85. Fagan RP, Albesa-Jove D, Qazi O, et al. Structural insights into the molecular organization of the S-layer from Clostridium difficile. Mol Microbiol 2009;71: 1308–22.
86. Ryan A, Lynch M, Smith SM, et al. A role for TLR4 in Clostridium difficile infection and the recognition of surface layer proteins. PLoS Pathog 2011;7:e1002076.
87. Eidhin DB, O'Brien JB, McCabe MS, et al. Active immunization of hamsters against Clostridium difficile infection using surface-layer protein. FEMS Immunol Med Microbiol 2008;52:207–18.
88. Tasteyre A, Karjalainen T, Avesani V, et al. Phenotypic and genotypic diversity of the flagellin gene (fliC) among Clostridium difficile isolates from different serogroups. J Clin Microbiol 2000;38:3179–86.
89. Tasteyre A, Karjalainen T, Avesani V, et al. Molecular characterization of fliD gene encoding flagellar cap and its expression among Clostridium difficile isolates from different serogroups. J Clin Microbiol 2001;39:1178–83.
90. Pechine S, Janoir C, Boureau H, et al. Diminished intestinal colonization by Clostridium difficile and immune response in mice after mucosal immunization with surface proteins of Clostridium difficile. Vaccine 2007;25:3946–54.
91. Ganeshapillai J, Vinogradov E, Rousseau J, et al. Clostridium difficile cell-surface polysaccharides composed of pentaglycosyl and hexaglycosyl phosphate repeating units. Carbohydr Res 2008;343:703–10.
92. Oberli MA, Hecht ML, Bindschadler P, et al. A possible oligosaccharide-conjugate vaccine candidate for Clostridium difficile is antigenic and immunogenic. Chem Biol 2011;18:580–8.
93. Monteiro MA, Ma Z, Bertolo L, et al. Carbohydrate-based Clostridium difficile vaccines. Expert Rev Vaccines 2013;12:421–31.
94. Pizarro-Guajardo M, Olguin-Araneda V, Barra-Carrasco J, et al. Characterization of the collagen-like exosporium protein, BclA1, of Clostridium difficile spores. Anaerobe 2013;25:18–30.
95. Lawley TD, Croucher NJ, Yu L, et al. Proteomic and genomic characterization of highly infectious Clostridium difficile 630 spores. J Bacteriol 2009;191:5377–86.
96. Cox AD, St Michael F, Aubry A, et al. Investigating the candidacy of a lipoteichoic acid-based glycoconjugate as a vaccine to combat Clostridium difficile infection. Glycoconj J 2013;30:843–55.

Predictive Values of Models of *Clostridium difficile* Infection

Caroline H. Chilton, PhD[a],*, Jane Freeman, PhD[b]

KEYWORDS

- *Clostridium difficile* infection • Animal model • *In vitro* model

KEY POINTS

- Animal and *in vitro* models continue to be valuable in understanding of *Clostridium difficile* infection (CDI).
- All available models of CDI have limitations, which may affect their predictive value.
- An understanding of model limitations is key when interpreting data.
- Use of different models can improve predictability.

CLOSTRIDIUM DIFFICILE AND THE NEED FOR MODELS

CDI remains a significant burden on hospitals and health care facilities worldwide. It is estimated that the incremental cost associated with CDI ranges from £4577 to £8843 across Europe[1] and from $4846 to $8570 in the United States.[2] The production of hardy spores is key, allowing persistence in both the hospital environment, creating a reservoir of infection, and in the gut, leading to recurrence and symptomatic relapse. Despite recent reductions in CDI incidence in some countries, the emergence of hypervirulent *C difficile* strains and a relative lack of therapeutic options mean that the organism remains a priority for health care institutions.

Pseudomembranous colitis (PMC) as a sequela of antibiotic use has been cited in the medical literature since the early 1950s.[3] It was not until the 1970s, however, that the search for an associated transmissible agent gained impetus, when Bartlett and colleagues[4] demonstrated the link between a toxin-producing species of clostridia and clindamycin-associated colitis in hamsters. Since then, animal models have been widely used in the study of CDI. Researchers have also used *in vitro* systems that circumvent some of the practical, ethical, and financial drawbacks of using animal

[a] Section of Molecular Gastroenterology, Leeds Institute for Biomedical and Clinical Sciences, University of Leeds, Old Medical School, Thoresby Place, Leeds LS1 3EX, UK; [b] Department of Microbiology, Leeds Teaching Hospitals NHS Trust, The General Infirmary, Old Medical School, Thoresby Place, Leeds LS1 3EX, UK
* Corresponding author.
E-mail address: c.h.chilton@leeds.ac.uk

Infect Dis Clin N Am 29 (2015) 163–177
http://dx.doi.org/10.1016/j.idc.2014.11.011
0891-5520/15/$ – see front matter © 2015 Elsevier Inc. All rights reserved.

models. Both *in vivo* and *in vitro* studies have been invaluable tools in the study of CDI. They offer several advantages over clinical studies, such as standardization of disease severity, flexibility to perform invasive tests and tissue sampling, and the capability to evaluate novel treatments. Model studies are unaffected by lack of available subjects and are not subject to the constraints of recruitment criteria, which can affect the success of some clinical studies. Lack of capability of some animal models to accurately mimic some aspects of *C difficile* pathogenesis, however, such as recurrent disease, or to generate reflective immune responses is a key limitation. This review examines the contribution and predictive value of both animal and *in vitro* models to CDI research.

EXISTING MODELS FOR *CLOSTRIDIUM DIFFICILE* INFECTION
Animal Models

An array of animal models has been used for the study of CDI, some more extensively than others. The most widely used are the hamster and mouse, and these are discussed in more detail. Guinea pigs, piglets, hares, rats, rabbits, prairie dogs, foals, rhesus monkeys, and zebra fish embryos have also been used in the study of *C difficile*, but a detailed discussion is beyond the scope of this article and readers are directed to the reviews by Best and colleagues[5] and Hutton and colleagues[6] for a more complete evaluation.

The hamster model was established as a model of CDI in the 1970s.[7,8] Studies[4,9–11] using the hamster model demonstrated a link between clindamycin-induced enterocolitis and a toxin-producing species of clostridia, paving the way for the identification of *C difficile* as the etiologic agent of PMC and implicating it in antibiotic-associated diarrhea. The contribution of the hamster model to understanding of CDI is considerable. CDI is a multifactorial disease, and this is reflected in the breadth of studies performed in the hamster model. Colonization resistance, inducing antibiotics; novel treatments; immunologic responses; and the action of toxins are some of those examined. Hamsters are acutely susceptible, however, to *C difficile* and do not necessarily exhibit diarrhea—a key feature of the disease in humans. The extreme susceptibility of the golden Syrian hamster to *C difficile* probably expedited the discovery of the organism as the etiologic agent of PMC but is ironically now seen as one of its major drawbacks. After induction of CDI with clindamycin, it is rapidly fatal. Therefore, the hamster model is actually a prevention of death model, with the endpoint being survival in days. This presents ethical problems, and in many countries animal welfare legislation requires the animals be euthanized. In addition, at a time when interest in the use of vaccines for *C difficile* is increasing, the hamster model is limited by a lack of immunologic tools with which to study host response.

Recent years have seen an increase in the use of mice as CDI models. These have been able to overcome some of the problems inherent in the hamster model (ie, poor reflection of human disease process and rapid fatality) and researchers also benefit from a wide availability of immunologic tools. Germfree mice exhibit many of the symptoms observed in the course of human CDI, such as diarrhea, lethargy, weight loss, and gut histologic changes, and have the advantage of needing no prior antibiotic treatment to elicit symptomatic disease.[12,13] Recently, mice have been used to examine other factors relevant to CDI, such as *C difficile* transcriptome during disease[14] and mapping of cecal and colonic cytokines.[12] Although gnotobiotic mouse models are well suited to study of the organism's direct interaction with its host, they lack a host microflora, and, therefore, some associated mucosal and immune responses are not present.[15]

Chen and colleagues[16] used a cocktail of antibiotics to disrupt the normal flora of C57BL/6 mice prior to *C difficile* exposure. The use of single CDI-inducing agents in small animal models has also been popular.[17–21] Certain antibiotics (clindamycin and cephalosporins) are associated with increased risk of CDI in humans. Therefore, use of a single inducing antibiotic allows the risk of CDI, specific action on the gut flora, and disease development to be assessed. Models that use a single antibiotic to induce CDI are more likely, however, to be influenced by variations in gut flora and antimicrobial susceptibility between mice from different sources. Antibiotic cocktail models may give a more consistent and reproducible degree of gut flora perturbation. Both single-agent and antibiotic cocktail mouse models exhibit CDI symptoms similar to those in humans: diarrhea, weight loss, and histologic damage. Chen and colleagues[16] also used varying spore doses or different *C difficile* strains to elicit the full spectrum of disease and, importantly, induction of symptomatic recurrences in mice that recovered from primary infection.

Small animal models have associated issues of environmental and cross-contamination, and coprophagia. All these factors may influence the extent of *C difficile* exposure and thus experimental outcome. Retrospective interexperimental comparisons (especially of early studies) are hampered by a lack of information regarding the introduction of *C difficile* to the animals and by the different antimicrobial doses and administration routes. Clindamycin has usually been the agent of choice when inducing CDI in animal models. There is significant variation, however, in the dose (ranging from 1 to 100 mg/kg).[5] *C difficile* exposure was also poorly controlled and sometimes left to chance, but even in later studies the timing of *C difficile* exposure and the inoculum preparation may differ considerably. More recent small animal experiments have recognized the need for strict environmental control, sterility protocols, and dosing regimens, particularly for the highly susceptible hamster model. Douce and Goulding[22] recommended individual housing in sterile cages and use of sterile food, water, and bedding plus daily transfer to a newly sterile environment.

In Vitro Models

Borriello and Barclay[23] pioneered the use of *in vitro* fecal emulsion models to describe the importance of the normal gut microflora in prevention of CDI. They also compared the fecal emulsion model with the hamster model to ascertain its predictive value, showing a high degree of correlation between the two. Similar batch culture investigations have been performed using cecal contents of mice.[24] Several groups have used batch culture fecal/cecal emulsion models to evaluate the effects of various antimicrobials on colonization resistance and CDI growth.[24–26] Their results, however, have not always reflected those seen clinically.[26]

Simple batch culture models do not accurately reflect the *in vivo* gut environments, whose growth dynamics are better reflected in continuous culture systems. Several groups reported conflicting results in simple batch culture investigations of antimicrobial effects on fecal emulsions.[27,28] Such approaches do not they lend themselves to the study of more recent areas of interest, such as disease recurrence, transmission, or restoration of gut flora. Consequently, researchers have developed more complex continuous culture systems. In addition to clear ethical advantages over animal models, they bring the additional benefits of longer experimental courses, multiple sampling points, and high degree of environmental manipulation and control. Onderdonk and colleagues[29] were the first to describe the development of a continuous culture method for *C difficile* and used this model to show that changes in redox potential (Eh) and temperature and subinhibitory levels of antimicrobials all increased levels of *C difficile* toxin production.

More recently, a triple-stage continuous culture *in vitro* model of CDI has been developed[30] and used in an extensive series of experiments to investigate the propensity of antimicrobials to induce simulated CDI (vegetative *C difficile* growth and corresponding toxin production),[31–33] and the efficacy of CDI treatments.[34–41] This model allows investigation of antimicrobial effects on gut microflora, *C difficile* germination and toxin production, recurrence, and intestinal biofilm. Effects can be monitored for longer periods than in animal or batch culture models. This model allows controlled and reproducible simulation of disease after instillation of an inducing antimicrobial (**Fig. 1**) and can be used to investigate recurrent disease. **Table 1** summarizes some of the advantages and disadvantages of *in vivo* and *in vitro* models.

USE OF MODELS TO INVESTIGATE DISEASE SEVERITY AND MECHANISMS

The elucidation of CDI as a toxin-mediated disease led to several studies examining the effects of toxins A and B in the hamster model.[42–44] Although early studies indicated that toxin A was more important than toxin B, later investigations in the hamster model have reasserted the role of both toxins in CDI pathogenesis.[45] The hamster

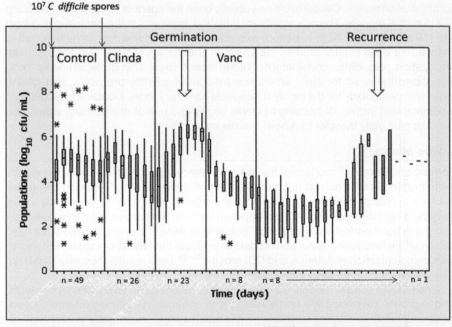

Fig. 1. Collated data from a triple-stage gut model of CDI showing box plots (median, interquartile ranges) of total *C difficile* population numbers ($\log_{10}$ colony-forming units [cfu]/mL) at different experimental stages. The number of models (n) in the analysis ranges from 49, which underwent a control period, down to 26, which received clindamycin, 8 that were treated with vancomycin, and, due to differences in the observation period after vancomycin instillation, this decreases over the displayed time frame. During the control period, *C difficile* spores are added without antimicrobial therapy and no germination occurs. A second aliquot of spores is added at the start of the clindamycin instillation period (Clinda). An increase in population numbers corresponds with germination, and populations subsequently decrease during and after vancomycin instillation (Vanc). Subsequent increases in population levels are indicative of recurrent disease.

Table 1
Summary of the main advantages and disadvantages of different *Clostridium difficile* infection models

	Human Fecal Emulsion	Hamster Cecal Emulsion	Continuous Culture (Gut Model)	Hamster Model	Mouse Model
Ethical and legal requirements	Minor ethical requirements	Significant ethical and legal issues to obtain hamster cecal contents	Minor ethical requirements	Significant ethical and legal issues	Significant ethical and legal issues
Practical requirements	Simple, inexpensive	Requires substantial equipment outlay and expertise Requires animal care in highly controlled environment Simple and inexpensive once cecal emulsion obtained	Requires substantial equipment outlay and expertise Labor-intensive sampling	Requires substantial equipment outlay and expertise Requires animal care in highly controlled environment to prevent accidental infection/reinfection and coprophagia Lack of immunologic tools	Requires substantial equipment outlay and expertise Requires animal care in highly controlled environment to prevent accidental infection/reinfection and coprophagia Readily available immunologic tools
Reflective of human disease	Germination and toxin production in antibiotic-containing emulsions Cannot model disease pathology or symptoms	Germination and toxin production in antibiotic-containing emulsions Cannot model disease pathology or symptoms	Germination and toxin production in response to predisposing antibiotics Cannot model disease pathology or symptoms	Does not wholly reflect human disease Diarrhea not always present Acutely susceptible; disease is rapidly fatal	Reflects human disease
Gut microflora	Batch culture not reflective of gut environment	Batch culture not reflective of gut environment	Gut reflective	Gut flora not necessarily reflective of human microflora	Gut flora not necessarily reflective of human microflora
Host responses	Cannot model host immunologic responses or secretory events	Cannot model host immunologic responses or secretory events	Cannot model host immunologic responses or secretory events	Host responses not necessarily reflective of human situation	Host responses not necessarily reflective of human situation
Other	Limited time course and, therefore, observations	Limited time course and, therefore, observations	Extensive time course, multiple observations Highly manipulable Able to model recurrence Able to model biofilm	Prevention of death model: difficult to study certain aspects of disease (eg relapse, transmission)	Able to model recurrence and transmission

model has been used investigate virulence of different *C difficile* strains.[46–49] Razaq and colleagues[50] demonstrated more rapid time to death from colonization with epidemic hypervirulent NAP1/BI strains. Warny and colleagues[51] described increased toxin production by *C difficile* NAP1 strains in *in vitro* batch culture. In a triple-stage gut model, however, this *C difficile* ribotype produces toxin for longer periods of time than comparator strains rather than increased peak levels.[41] Such differences in results highlight how models can markedly affect assumptions of disease pathogenesis and possibly show the advantage of using complex, continuous model systems rather than batch culture. Control of *C difficile* exposure has been variable in some studies, and infective dose is an important issue when determining the relative virulence to *C difficile* strains. The hamster model has notably been used to show the potential of nontoxigenic strains to prevent colonization by toxigenic *C difficile*.[52,53]

USE OF MODELS TO INVESTIGATE COLONIZATION RESISTANCE

The protective value of the normal gut flora, termed 'colonization resistance', is a major area of research. Disruption of normal flora by antimicrobial action is thought to play a significant role in CDI development. Repopulation of the gut microflora by fecal transplantation has been clinically effective in treating CDI and preventing recurrent disease. Early fecal emulsion models reflected this, demonstrating that feces from healthy adults inhibited growth and toxin production of *C difficile*, whereas samples that were sterilized by filtration or autoclaving did not. The investigators attributed this colonization resistance to viable components within the fecal emulsion of healthy individuals.[23] The fecal emulsion model was compared with the hamster model to ascertain its predictive value, showing a high degree of correlation,[23] and similar investigations have been performed using cecal contents of mice.[24] Colonization resistance is also reflected in continuous culture systems. Wilson and Freter[54] investigated the interactions between the entire fecal flora of hamsters and *C difficile* (and *Escherichia coli*) in gnotobiotic mice and a continuous-flow culture system.[55] In both *in vivo* and *in vitro* models, hamster cecal flora suppressed potential pathogens, the *C difficile* population decreased, and the addition of the continuous culture contents decreased the size of the germfree mouse ceca back to normal. In the more complex triple-stage gut model, simulated CDI does not occur until after antimicrobial instillation.[34,35]

Several antibiotic mouse models have contributed to this area of interest. Lawley and colleagues[18] were able to demonstrate that mice exposed to epidemic strains of *C difficile* developed relapsing disease that was refractile to vancomycin treatment and showed distinct and simplified (less diverse) fecal flora. Treatment with feces of healthy mice rapidly restored the microflora to that of a healthy mouse and the disease was resolved.[18] This raises the possibility of using antibiotic mouse models for the investigation of fecal microbiota transplantation.

USE OF MODELS TO INVESTIGATE INDUCTION OF *CLOSTRIDIUM DIFFICILE* INFECTION

Early work on the relative predisposition of various antimicrobials was performed in the hamster model but hampered by lack of standardization.[5] Larson and Borriello[55] were the first to tackle this by standardizing the *C difficile* strain and inoculum and housing hamsters in a sterile environment. Using this improved model, the investigators demonstrated that clindamycin induced a much greater window of susceptibility to CDI than other antibiotics and suggested that antibiotics may differ in terms of relative CDI risk.[56] Since then, further improvements in the control of animal environments have been recommended.[22]

Almost all classes of antimicrobials have been associated with the induction of CDI. Clindamycin, third-generation cephalosporins, and aminopenicillins have been commonly associated with the disease since the 1980s, and fluoroquinolones have more recently emerged as higher risk agents for CDI.[57] Several comparative studies have investigated antibiotic induction of CDI in both *in vivo* and *in vitro* models. There has been broad agreement between animal and *in vitro* models with respect to clindamycin,[34–41] aminopenicillins, and third-generation cephalosporins.[30,56,58,59] Likewise, the more recent attribution of CDI risk to fluoroquinolones has been reflected in hamsters[60] and in gut model studies[61]; both approaches highlight the possible relationship between fluoroquinolone resistance in epidemic *C difficile* strain and the emergence of increased CDI risk for these agents. Determination of the CDI induction risk of piperacillin/tazobactam has been less clear. Piperacillin/tazobactam is considered low risk for CDI in humans.[57,62] but *C difficile* growth and toxin production was reported in piperacillin-treated mouse cecal emulsions[26] and shown to induce colitis in hamsters.[63] Contrastingly, piperacillin/tazobactam did not elicit germination and toxin production in a more complex triple-stage chemostat gut model.[32]

Both animal and *in vitro* models have indicated a potential role for *C difficile* susceptibility in the timing of germination and toxin production. Gut model studies have indicated that germination and toxin production by *C difficile* occur when the inducing drug concentration falls below the minimum inhibitory concentration of the strain.[34–37,39,41] Similar observations have also been made in hamsters.[57,64] Although, the fecal/cecal emulsion model is considered an *in vitro* CDI model, the test antimicrobials have been administered to and metabolized by an animal. Therefore, the caveats attendant on the use of animal models (ie, potentially different host microflora, immune responses, and metabolism of compounds) may also hold true.

USE OF MODELS TO EVALUATE EFFICACY OF EXISTING AND NOVEL *CLOSTRIDIUM DIFFICILE* INFECTION TREATMENTS

Evaluation of treatment efficacy is achieved ultimately by randomized controlled clinical trials; however, preliminary indications, such as efficacy in models, are required before expensive clinical trials can be justified (see **Table 1**). Hence, the understanding of the predictive value of models in terms of evaluation of novel treatment agents is of key importance. They can provide important data on dosage, the effect of the agent on *C difficile* itself (ie, any antispore effects), likely effects on gut flora and the duration thereof, and likelihood of recurrence. In cases of immunologic treatments, animal models can provide data on host response. Caution must be taken, however, when interpreting animal model data, because immunologic responses vary between animals.[65]

Vancomycin and metronidazole have been the CDI treatment drugs of choice for many years,[66] with the former agent identified as an effective treatment of antibiotic-associated pseudomembranous enterocolitis even before *C difficile* was identified as its cause.[67] High rates of recurrence observed, however, after vancomycin and metronidazole,[68] reports of reduced susceptibility to metronidazole,[69] recent evidence questioning the efficacy of metronidazole,[70] and the high costs associated with fidaxomicin (the only novel approved CDI treatment)[71] combine to ensure the search for novel treatment agents continues.

A variety of models have been used to glean information on the efficacy of treatment agents (as discussed in **Table 2**), although the concordance with clinical data has been variable. For fidaxomicin, data from animal and *in vitro* models correlated well with phase III clinical trials.[38,76,78] By contrast, for the toxin-binding agent, tolevamer,

Table 2
Summary of data on efficacy of treatment agents gather using different models

Treatment Agent	Data from Animal Models	Data from In Vitro Models	Clinical Data
Metronidazole	• In hamster model, prevents fatal antibiotic-induced colitis during instillation[7,72] • After instillation, fatal colitis can ensue. 20% survival rate 14 d postinstillation[72]	• Ineffective in resolving simulated CDI in the triple-stage gut model with no effect on vegetative cell growth or toxin production for polymerase chain reaction ribotype 027 strains[38,41] • Possible inactivation of metronidazole by gut microflora observed[38,41,73]	• Considered for many years to be noninferior to vancomycin for treatment of initial infection[68,74] and first recurrence[75] • More recently shown inferior to vancomycin in randomized controlled clinical trials ($P = .02$),[71] although rate of recurrence similar to vancomycin
Vancomycin	• Hamster model first used to demonstrate efficacy of vancomycin for prevention of clindamycin-induced colitis[4,7,76,77]	• Successfully resolves simulated CDI in triple-stage gut model (see **Fig. 1**)[35,36,38,40,59] • Recurrence of vegetative cell growth and toxin production observed in some cases,[35,38] but not others,[40] which may be due to length of postinstillation observation time	• Identified as successful treatment of antibiotic-associated pseudomembranous enterocolitis even before C difficile was identified as the causative agent[67] • Generally used as the comparator in clinical trials. Good efficacy in treatment of CDI[70,78–80] • Recurrence rates of ~20%[68]
Fidaxomicin	• In hamster model, administration of 0.2, 1, or 5 mg per kg body weight resulted 100% survival of clindamycin treated hamsters exposed to C difficile ATCC 968. Indicated superiority of fidaxomicin to vancomycin[76]	• Rapidly reduced vegetative cells, spore counts and toxin production in the triple-stage gut model with no sign of recurrence[38] • Prevented recovery of spores for long periods of time, unlike vancomycin[38] • Persistence of antimicrobial activity observed[38] • Preserved the microbiome (except bifidobacteria)[38]	• Noninferior to vancomycin for initial clinical cure in two phase III randomized controlled trials[79,80] • Superior to vancomycin in prevention of recurrence[78] • High concentrations and persistence of activity in stool observed[81,82] • Preserved the microbiome (including bifidobacteria)[83]

Tolevamer	• Effective in treatment of antibiotic-induced colitis in hamsters, protecting 80% from mortality[72] • No dose dependence noted in hamster model[72] • Withdrawal of tolevamer did not lead to relapse[72]	• Ineffective in neutralizing toxin in the triple-stage gut model, which continued to be detected at pretreatment levels[34]	• In phase II trials, successfully resolved diarrhea in 83% patients (6 g/d) compared with 93% receiving vancomycin Shown noninferior to vancomycin with a trend toward lower rates of recurrence[84] • In phase III randomized controlled trials, however, tolevamer was inferior to both vancomycin and metronidazole.[70] • Inferior in treatment of severe CDI, although this did not reach statistical significance ($P = .059$)[70]
Cadazolid	• Dose-dependant protective effect observed in the mouse model, with 100% survival at day 5 and 88% survival at day 18[77] • Protective in hamster model during treatment but with varying degrees of post-treatment survival[77]	• Two different dosing regimens (250 or 750 mg/L, twice daily, 7 d) rapidly resolved simulated CDI in the gut model[37]	• Clinical efficacy recently demonstrated in phase II clinical trials[85]
Surotomycin	• Instillation conferred complete protection against antibiotic-induced colitis in hamsters[86] • Time- and dose-dependant postantibiotic effect observed, with hamsters beginning to succumb to colitis from 6 d postinstillation[86]	• Rapidly resolved simulated CDI caused by 2 different polymerase chain reaction ribotype strains in the triple-stage gut model[39] • Recurrence of vegetative *C difficile* growth and toxin production observed 11–15 d after cessation of instillation.[39]	• No inferiority to vancomycin for initial clinical cure demonstrated in phase II clinical trials[54] • Higher rate of sustained clinical cure and delayed time to recurrence observed compared with vancomyin[54]
Fecal microbiota transplant	• Microbiota of mice infected with *C difficile* distinct and simplified from healthy mice Transplantation of feces from a healthy mouse returned microbiota to normal and resolved disease symptoms.[18] • A cocktail of 6 organisms, which had the same effect as healthy mouse feces was also identified.[18] • Cecal flora from hamsters suppressed *C difficile* in gnotobiotic mice.[55]	• *In vitro* batch culture showed that healthy fecal slurries prevented *C difficile* growth and toxin production, whereas feces from *C difficile* infected patients did not.[23] • Cecal content of mice suppressed *C difficile* growth in batch culture.[24] • Cecal flora of hamsters prevented *C difficile* growth in a continuous culture system.[55]	• A small clinical trial in patients demonstrated that fecal transplant resolved *C difficile*–associated diarrhea in 83% of patients compared with 31% of patients receiving vancomycin alone, and 23% receiving vancomycin with bowel lavage.[87]

animal model data did not correlate with the results of phase III trial where the drug performed poorly[70,72]; results from a triple-stage gut model predicted that tolevamer may not be effective *in vivo*.[34] Although the gut model is an effective and apparently predictive means of evaluating potential anti-CDI treatments, it cannot provide the observations generated by multiple subjects in a clinical trial.

CLOSTRIDIUM DIFFICILE INFECTION RECURRENCE IN MODELS

A key area in recent *C difficile* research is the issue of disease recurrence. In humans, a relatively high proportion of patients (up to 20%–30%)[68] suffer from symptomatic recurrences. This has become an important consideration in the differentiation of potential CDI therapeutics. Symptomatic recurrence is due either to germination of residual *C difficile* spores after antimicrobial therapy or reacquisition of *C difficile* from the environment. Symptomatic recurrence and *C difficile* carriage are difficult to study in hamsters because of their acute susceptibility to and poor rate of recovery from CDI. After cessation of instillation of treatment agents, however, development of colitis can be seen.[77] Often this is due to post-treatment acquisition of *C difficile* (reinfection).[88] Fatal colitis has been observed after cessation of both vancomycin[7,77] and metronidazole.[7,72]

CDI recurrence has been more successfully modeled in mice. Lawley and colleagues[18] were able to demonstrate symptomatic recurrences in their clindamycin mouse model, showing that in contrast to other *C difficile* strains, infection with epidemic ribotype 027 induces a supershedder state leading to enhanced transmission. The gut model has also been used to successfully simulate recurrence after vancomcyin treatment.[38] Typically, recurrence (*C difficile* germination and toxin production) is observed approximately 12 to 14 days after the cessation of vancomycin instillation (see **Fig. 1**), and detection is dependent on the length of the postantibiotic observation period.[39] The host immune response, however, likely influences risk of CDI recurrence. *In vitro* systems typically lack key host response factors. Similarly, host immune response in animal models may not be reflective of human immune responses.

SUMMARY

Both animal and *in vitro* models have made valuable contributions to the understanding of CDI and continue to do so in many areas of research. All available models of CDI have limitations, however, which may affect their predictive value. An understanding of these limitations is, therefore, key when interpreting model data. Use of a variety of approaches can improve understanding of the disease and the predictability of responses to interventions. Development of novel models more able to accurately mimic the human immune system may be required in novel areas of research, such as vaccine development and antibody therapy. To this extent, the recent use of stem cell–derived human intestinal organoids to examine *C difficile* behavior is noted.[89] Such novel models could potentially be exploited to address unanswered questions surrounding the pathogenesis of CDI.

REFERENCES

1. Wiegand PN, Nathwani D, Wilcox MH, et al. Clinical and economic burden of Clostridium difficile infection in Europe: a systematic review of healthcare-facility-acquired infection. J Hosp Infect 2012;81:1–14.

2. Ghantoji SS, Sail K, Lairson DR, et al. Economic healthcare costs of Clostridium difficile infection: a systematic review. J Hosp Infect 2010;74:309–18.
3. Reiner L, Schlesinger MJ, Miller GM. Pseudomembranous colitis following aureomycin and chloramphenicol. AMA Arch Pathol 1952;54(1):39–67.
4. Bartlett JG, Onderdonk AB, Cisneros RL. Clindamycin-associated colitis in hamsters: protection with vancomycin. Gastroenterology 1977;73:772–6.
5. Best EL, Freeman J, Wilcox MH. Models for the study of Clostridium difficile infection. Gut Microbes 2012;3:145–67.
6. Hutton ML, Mackin KE, Chakravorty A, et al. Small animal models for the study of Clostridium difficile disease pathogenesis. FEMS Microbiol Lett 2014;352:140–9.
7. Fekety R, Silva J, Toshniwal R, et al. Antibiotic-associated colitis: effects of antibiotics on Clostridium difficile and the disease in hamsters. Rev Infect Dis 1979;1:386–97.
8. Toshniwal R, Fekety R, Silva J. Etiology of tetracycline-associated pseudomembranous colitis in hamsters. Antimicrob Agents Chemother 1979;16:167–70.
9. Bartlett JG, Chang TW, Moon N, et al. Antibiotic-induced lethal enterocolitis in hamsters: studies with eleven agents and evidence to support the pathogenic role of toxin-producing Clostridia. Am J Vet Res 1978;39(9):1525–30.
10. Bartlett JG. Antimicrobial agents implicated in Clostridium difficile toxin-associated diarrhea of colitis. Johns Hopkins Med J 1981;149:6–9.
11. Rifkin GD, Silva J, Fekety R. Gastrointestinal and systemic toxicity of fecal extracts from hamsters with clindamycin-induced colitis. Gastroenterology 1978;74:52–7.
12. Pawlowski SW, Calarese G, Kolling GL. Murine model of Clostridium difficile infection with aged gnotobiotic C57BL/6 mice and a BI/NAP1 strain. J Infect Dis 2010;202:1708–12.
13. Reeves AE, Koenigsknecht MJ, Bergin IL, et al. Suppression of Clostridium difficile in the gastronintestinal tracts of germfree mice inoculated with a murine isolate from the family Lachnospiraceae. Infect Immun 2012;80:3786–94.
14. Janoir C, Deneve C, Bouuttier S, et al. Adaptive strategies and pathogenesis of Clostridium difficile from in vivo transcriptomics. Infect Immun 2013;81:3757–89.
15. Macpherson AJ, Harris NL. Interactions between commensal intestinal bacteria and the immune system. Nat Rev Immunol 2004;4:478–785.
16. Chen X, Katchar K, Goldsmith JD, et al. A mouse model of Clostridium difficile-associated disease. Gastroenterology 2008;135:1984–92.
17. Lawley TD, Clare S, Walker AW, et al. Antibiotic treament of Clostridium difficile carrier mice triggers a supershedder state, spore-mediated transmission, and severe disease in immunocompromised hosts. Infect Immun 2009;77:3661–9.
18. Lawley TD, Clare S, Walker AW, et al. Targeted restoration of the intestinal microbiota with a simple, defined bacteriotherapy resolves relapsing Clostridium difficile disease in mice. PLoS Pathog 2012;8:e1002995.
19. Buffie CG, Jarchum I, Equinda M, et al. Profound alterations of intestinal microbiota following a single dose of clindamycin results in sustained susceptibility to Clostridium difficile-induced colitis. Infect Immun 2012;80:62–73.
20. Theriot CM, Koumpouras CC, Carlson PE, et al. Cefoperazone-treated mice asan experimental platform to assess differential virulence of Clostridium difficile strains. Gut Microbes 2011;2:326 34.
21. Sun X, Wang H, Zhang Y, et al. Mouse relapse model of Clostridium difficile infection. Infect Immun 2011;79:2856–64.
22. Douce G, Goulding D. Refinement of the hamster mode of Clostridium difficile disease. Methods Mol Biol 2010;646:215–27.

23. Borriello SP, Barclay FE. An in vitro model of colonization resistance to clostridium difficile infection. J Med Microbiol 1986;21:299–309.
24. Adams DA, Riggs MM, Donskey CJ. Effect of fluoroquinolone treatment on growth of and toxin production by epidemic and nonepidemic clostridium difficile strains in the cecal contents of mice. Antimicrob Agents Chemother 2007;51: 2674–8.
25. Jump RL, LI Y, Pultz MJ, et al. Tigecycline exhibits inhibitory activity against Clostridium difficile in the colon of mice and does not promote growth or toxin production. Antimicrob Agents Chemother 2011;55:546–9.
26. Pultz NJ, Donskey CJ. Effect of antibiotic treatment on growth of and toxin production by Clostridium difficile in the cecal contents of mice. Antimicrob Agents Chemother 2005;49:3529–32.
27. Drummond LJ, Smith DG, Poxton IR. Effects of sub-MIC concentrations of antibiotics on growth and toxin production by Clostridium difficile. J Med Microbiol 2003;52:1033–8.
28. Barc MC, Depitre C, Corthier G, et al. Effects of antibiotics and other drugs on toxin production in Clostridium difficile in vitro and in vivo. Antimicrob Agents Chemother 1992;36:1332–5.
29. Onderdonk AB, Lowe BR, Bartlett JG. Effect of environmental stress on Clostridium difficile toxin levels during continuous cultivation. Appl Environ Microbiol 1979;8:637–41.
30. Freeman J, O'Neill FJ, Wilcox MH. Effects of cefotaxime and desacetylcefotaxime upon Clostridium difficile proliferation and toxin production in a triple-stage chemostat model of the human gut. J Antimicrob Chemother 2003;52:96–102.
31. Baines SD, Chilton CH, Crowther GS, et al. Evaluation of antimicrobial activity of ceftaroline against Clostridium difficile and propensity to induce C-difficile infection in an in vitro human gut model. J Antimicrob Chemother 2013;68:1842–9.
32. Baines SD, Freeman J, Wilcox MH. Effects of piperacillin/tazobactam on Clostridium difficile growth and toxin production in a human gut model. J Antimicrob Chemother 2005;55:974–82.
33. Chilton CH, Freeman J, Crowther GS, et al. Co-amoxiclav induces proliferation and cytotoxin production of Clostridium difficile ribotype 027 in a human gut model. J Antimicrob Chemother 2012;67:951–4.
34. Baines SD, Freeman J, Wilcox MH. Tolevamer is not efficacious in the neutralization of cytotoxin in a human gut model of Clostridium difficile infection. Antimicrob Agents Chemother 2009;53:2202–4.
35. Baines SD, O'Connor R, Saxton K, et al. Comparison of oritavancin versus vancomycin as treatments for clindamycin-induced Clostridium difficile PCR ribotype 027 infection in a human gut model. J Antimicrob Chemother 2008;62:1078–85.
36. Baines SD, O'Connor R, Saxton K, et al. Activity of vancomycin against epidemic Clostridium difficile strains in a human gut model. J Antimicrob Chemother 2009; 63:520–5.
37. Chilton CH, Crowther GS, Baines SD, et al. In vitro activity of cadazolid against clinically relevant Clostridium difficile isolates and in an in vitro gut model of C. difficile infection. J Antimicrob Chemother 2014;69:697–705.
38. Chilton CH, Crowther GS, Freeman J, et al. Successful treatment of simulated Clostridium difficile infection in a human gut model by fidaxomicin first line and after vancomycin or metronidazole failure. J Antimicrob Chemother 2014;69:451–62.
39. Chilton CH, Crowther GS, Todhunter SL, et al. Efficacy of surotomycin in an in vitro gut model of Clostridium difficile infection. J Antimicrob Chemother 2014;69: 2426–33.

40. Freeman J, Baines SD, Jabes D, et al. Comparison of the efficacy of ramoplanin and vancomycin in both in vitro and in vivo models of clindamycin-induced *Clostridium difficile* infection. J Antimicrob Chemother 2005;56:717–25.
41. Freeman J, Baines SD, Saxton K, et al. Effect of metronidazole on growth and toxin production by epidemic Clostridium difficile PCR ribotypes 001 and 027 in a human gut model. J Antimicrob Chemother 2007;60:83–91.
42. Taylor NS, Thorne GM, Bartlett JG. Comparison of two toxins produced by *Clostridium difficile*. Infect Immun 1981;34:1036–43.
43. Lyerly DM, Saum KE, Macdonald DK, et al. Effects of *Clostridium difficile* toxins given intragastrically to animals. Infect Immun 1985;47:349–52.
44. Voth DE, Ballard JD. *Clostridium difficile* toxins: mechanism of action and role in disease. Clin Microbiol Rev 2005;18:247–63.
45. Kuehne SA, Cartman ST, Heap JT, et al. The role of toxin A and toxin B in *Clostridium difficile* infection. Nature 2010;467(7316):711–3.
46. Borriello SP, Ketley JM, Mitchell TJ, et al. Clostridium difficile–a spectrum of virulence and analysis of putative virulence determinants in the hamster model of antibiotic-associated colitis. J Med Microbiol 1987;24(1):53–64.
47. Delmee M, Avesani V. Virulence of ten serogroups of *Clostridium difficile* in hamsters. J Med Microbiol 1990;33:85–90.
48. Sambol SP, Tang JK, Merrigan MM, et al. Infection of hamsters with epidemiologically important strains of *Clostridium difficile*. J Infect Dis 2001;183:1760–6.
49. Goulding D, Thompson H, Emerson J, et al. Distinctive profiles of infection and pathology in hamsters infected with *Clostridium difficile* strains 630 and B1. Infect Immun 2009;77:5478–85.
50. Razaq N, Sambol S, Nagaro K, et al. Infection of hamsters with historical and epidemic BI types of *Clostridium difficile*. J Infect Dis 2007;196:1813–9.
51. Warny M, Pepin J, Fang A, et al. Toxin production by and emerging strain of *Clostridium difficile* associated with outbreaks of severe disease in North America and Europe. Lancet 2005;366:1079–84.
52. Sambol SP, Merrigan MM, Tang JK, et al. Colonization for the prevention of *Clostridium difficile* in hamsters. J Infect Dis 2002;186:1781–9.
53. Merrigan MM, Sambol SO, Johnson S, et al. New approach to the management of *Clostridium difficile* infection: colonisation with non-toxigenic C. difficile during daily ampicillin or ceftriaxone adminisitration. Int J Antimicrob Agents 2009;33:S46–50.
54. Wilson KH, Freter R. Interaction of *Clostridium difficile* and *Escherichia coli* with microfloras in continuous-flow cultures and gnotobiotic mice. Infect Immun 1986;54:354–8.
55. Larson HE, Borriello SP. Quantitative study of antibiotic-induced susceptibility to *Clostridium difficile* enterocecitis in hamsters. Antimicrob Agents Chemother 1990;34:1348–53.
56. Slimings C, Riley TV. Antibiotics and hospital-acquired *Clostridium difficile* infection: update of systematic review and meta-analysis. J Antimicrob Chemother 2014;69:881–91.
57. Ebright JR, Fekety R, Silva J, et al. Evaluation of eight cephalosporins in hamster colitis model. Antimicrob Agents Chemother 1981;19(6):980–6.
58. Crowther GS, Baines SD, Todhunter SL, et al. Evaluation of NVB302 versus vancomycin activity in an in vitro human gut model of *Clostridium difficile* infection. J Antimicrob Chemother 2013;68:168–76.
59. Phillips ST, Nagaro K, Sambol SP, et al. Susceptibility of hamsters to infection by historic and epidemic BI *Clostridium difficile* strains during daily administration of three fluoroquinolones. Anaerobe 2011;17(4):166–9.

60. Saxton K, Baines SD, Freeman J, et al. Effects of exposure of *Clostridium difficile* PCR ribotypes 027 and 001 to fluoroquinolones in a human gut model. Antimicrob Agents Chemother 2009;53(2):412–20.

61. Settle CD, Wilcox MH, Fawley WN, et al. Prospective study of the risk of Clostridium difficile diarrhoea in elderly patients following treatment with cefotaxime or piperacillin-tazobactam. Aliment Pharmacol Ther 1998;12:1217–23.

62. Elmer GW, Vega R, Mohutsky MA, et al. Variable time of onset of Clostridium difficile disease initiated by antimicrobial treatment in hamsters. Microb Ecol Health Dis 1999;11:163–8.

63. Wilson KH, Silva J, Fekety FR. Suppression of *Clostridium difficile* by normal hamster cecal flora and prevention of antibiotic-associated cecitis. Infect Immun 1981;34:626–8.

64. Kyne L, Warney M, Qamar A, et al. Asymptomatic carriage of *Clostridium difficile* and serum levels of IgG antibody against toxin A. N Engl J Med 2000;342: 390–7.

65. Aslam S, Hamill RJ, Musher DM. Treatment of Clostridium difficile-associated disease: old therapies and new strategies. Lancet Infect Dis 2005;5(9):549–57.

66. Khan MY, Hall WH. Staphylococcal enterocolitis–treatment with oral vancomycin. Ann Intern Med 1966;65:1–8.

67. Wilcox MH, Fawley WN, Settle CD, et al. Recurrence of symptoms in *Clostridium difficile* infection–relapse or reinfection? J Hosp Infect 1998;38:93–100.

68. Baines SD, O'Connor R, Freeman J, et al. Emergence of reduced susceptibility to metronidazole in Clostridium difficile. J Antimicrob Chemother 2008;62(5): 1046–52.

69. Johnson S, Louie TJ, Gerding DN, et al. Vancomycin, metronidazole, or tolevamer for clostridium difficile infection: results from two multinational, randomized, controlled trials. Clin Infect Dis 2014;59(3):345–54.

70. Wagner M, Lavoie L, Goetghebeur M. Clinical and economic consequences of vancomycin and fidaxomicin for the treatment of Clostridium difficile infection in Canada. Can J Infect Dis Med Microbiol 2014;25(2):87–94.

71. Swanson RN, Hardy DJ, Shipkowitz NL, et al. In vitro and in vivo evaluation of tiacumicin-B and Tiacumicin-C against *Clostridium difficile*. Antimicrob Agents Chemother 1991;35:1108–11.

72. Locher HH, Seiler P, Chen X, et al. In vitro and in vivo antibacterial evaluation of cadazolid, a new antibiotic for treatment of *Clostridium difficile* infections. Antimicrob Agents Chemother 2014;58:892–900.

73. Gerding DN. Metronidazole for *Clostridium difficile*-associated disease: is it okay for Mom? Clin Infect Dis 2005;40:1598–600.

74. Pepin J, Routhier S, Gagnon S, et al. Management and outcomes of a first recurrence of *Clostridium difficile*-associated disease in Quebec, Canada. Clin Infect Dis 2006;42:758–64.

75. Louie TJ, Miller MA, Mullane KM, et al. Fidaxomicin versus vancomycin for *Clostridium difficile* infection. N Engl J Med 2011;364:422–31.

76. Crook DW, Walker AS, Kean Y, et al. Fidaxomicin versus vancomycin for *Clostridium difficile* infection: meta-analysis of pivotal randomized controlled trials. Clin Infect Dis 2012;55(Suppl 2):S93–103.

77. Fekety R, Silva J, Browne RA, et al. Clindamycin-induced colitis. Am J Clin Nutr 1979;32:244–50.

78. Kurtz CB, Connon EP, Brezzani A, et al. GT160-246, a toxin binding polymer for treatment of Clostridium difficile colitis. Antimicrob Agents Chemother 2001;45: 2340–7.

79. Cornely OA, Crook DW, Esposito R, et al. Fidaxomicin versus vancomycin for infection with Clostridium difficile in Europe, Canada, and the USA: a double-blind, non-inferiority, randomised controlled trial. Lancet Infect Dis 2012;12: 281–9.

80. Sears P, Crook DW, Louie TJ, et al. Fidaxomicin attains high fecal concentrations with minimal plasma concentrations following oral administration in patients with Clostridium difficile infection. Clin Infect Dis 2012;55(Suppl 2):S116–20.

81. European Medicines Agency. DIFICLIR Public Assessment Report. 2011. Available at: http://www.ema.europa.eu/docs/en_GB/document_library/EPAR_-_Public_assessment_report/human/002087/WC500119707.pdf. Accessed June 13, 2014.

82. Louie TJ, Connon K, Byrne B, et al. Fidaxomicin preserves the intestinal microbiome during and after treatment of *Clostridium difficile* infection (CDI) and reduces both toxin reexpression and recurrence of CDI. Clin Infect Dis 2012; 55(Suppl 2):S132–42.

83. Louie TJ, Peppe J, Watt CK, et al. Tolevamer, a novel nonantibiotic polymer, compared with vancomycin in the treatment of mild to moderately severe *Clostridium difficile* - Associated diarrhea. Clin Infect Dis 2006;43:411–20.

84. Louie T, Cornely OA, Kracker H, et al. Multicentre, double-blind, randomised, phase 2 study evaluating the novel antibiotic, cadazolid, in subjects with Clostridium difficile-associated diarrhoea. [Abtract LB-2956]. In: Programs and abstracts of the 23rd European Congress of clinical microbiology and Infectious Disease. Berlin, 27–30 April, 2013.

85. Mascio CT, Mortin LI, Howland KT, et al. In vitro and in vivo characterization of CB-183,315, a novel lipopeptide antibiotic for treatment of Clostridium difficile. Antimicrob Agents Chemother 2012;56:5023–30.

86. Pation HS, Stevens C, Louie T, et al. Efficacy and safety of the lipopeptide cb-183,315 for the treatment of clostridium difficile infection. [Abstract K-205a]. In: Programs and abstracts of the 51st Interscience Conference on Antimicrobial Agents and Chemotherapy. Chicago, 10–13 September, 2011. p. 278.

87. Van Nood E, Vrieze A, Nieuwdorp M, et al. Duodenal infusion of donor feces for recurrent Clostridium difficile. N Engl J Med 2013;368:407–15.

88. Nagy E, Foldes J. Inactivation of metronidazole by Enterococcus faecalis. J Antimicrob Chemother 1991;27:63–70.

89. Leslie JL, Huang S, Opp JS, et al. Persistence and toxin production by *Clostridium difficile* within human intestinal organoids results in disruption of epithelial paracellular barrier function. Infect Immun 2014. [Epub ahead of print].

Index

Note: Page numbers of article titles are in **boldface** type.

Printed and bound by CPI Group (UK) Ltd, Croydon, CR0 4YY

03/10/2024

01040488-0016